# YO
# A
# YOUR HEART

Hon. Brigadier (Late) **Dr. K.K. DATEY** SEM.
B.A., M.D., F.R.C.P.(LOND.), F.P.C.C. (Hon.), F.A.C.C.(U.S.A.),
F.A.M.S.(Ind), F.A.C.P. (Hon. U.S.A.), F.R.C.P. (Edin),
F.M.A.S.(Mah), F.R.S.A. (Lond.), F.C.H.S. (Can.), F.I.C.P.M.(Hol.),
D.C.H. (Eng.), F.A.A.B.S. (U.S.A.), F.N.A. (Ind.), D.T.M. & H.
(Lond.), F.C.C.P.(U.S.A.), F.I.C.A.(U.S.A.).

Director, Dept of Cardiology, Medical Resesarch Centre,
Bombay Hospital, Bombay.

Consultant in Cardiology, to the Armed Forces (Retd.) Professor
Emeritus, St. George's Hospital, BOMBAY

Consultant in Cardiology, Central Rly. Hq. Hospital, BOMBAY.

**DR. M. L. GHAROTE**
KAIVALYADHAMA, LONAVALA

(Late) **SOLI PAVRI**

Write
or
visit
for
books

## PRABHUS BOOKS
(A House of Books of your choice)
Ayurveda College Jn.,
Old Sreekanteswaram Road
Thiruvananthapuram - 695 001
Phone : 0471 - 478397, 473496

# JAICO PUBLISHING HOUSE
Mumbai • Delhi • Bangalore
Kolkata • Hyderabad • Chennai

YOGA AND YOUR HEART
ISBN 81-7224-032-5

Eigth Jaico Impression: 2002

Published by
Jaico Publishing House
121, Mahatma Gandhi Road,
Mumbai - 400 001

Printed by
Pramod Bhogate
Snehesh Printers
320-A, Shah & Nahar Ind.Est.- A-1,
Lower Parel, Mumbai - 400 013.

# CONTENTS

**Yogic Exercises**

# CONTENTS

# ACKNOWLEDGEMENTS

It is a great pleasure to acknowledge my gratitude to Dr. (Mrs.) S.J. BHAGAT, who helped in the preparation of this book. I also acknowledge my gratitude to Dr. K.R. SHARMA, Dr. ABBAS T. GHADIALY and Dr. ROHINTON A. CHHOGA for meticulously going through each sentence of the book and offering constructive and valuable suggestions. They have also been of immense help in the final proof-reading and preparation of the Index of this book.

## ACKNOWLEDGEMENTS

# PREFACE

Heart disease is spreading like an epidemic. In the United States of America, in 1925, cardiovascular disease accounted for 25% of all deaths, while in 1980 it accounts for over 50%. The incidence has more than doubled within less than half a century. In India, too, the incidence is on the increase. Our data from the city of Bombay shows that heart disease was the ninth cause of death in 1940, while in 1960 it became the third cause, headed only by infections and tuberculosis. As we all know, infections and tuberculosis can now be effectively controlled, and it will not be long before heart disease becomes the number one killer in India, too.

In India, about two decades ago heart attacks were rare in the younger age groups, but today, we are seeing patients between 30 and 40 years and even younger ones getting heart attacks. In the female sex, upto the age of 40, heart attacks were rare unless associated with risk factors. Now, even females are getting heart attacks between the ages of 30 and 40 years.

What are the causes of this epidemic of heart disease? The two important factors are tensions and diet. As compared with our forefathers, the tensions which modern man has to face have grown a hundred fold. As a result of mental tension, man is prone to smoke and drink so as to get a feeling of relaxation. He has, therefore, to resort to tranquillisers, sleeping pills, alcohol, tobacco etc. All this results in a sick mind. The body and mind have a close inter-relationship.

Our life-styles have changed and life-style includes the changes in our diet, lack of exercise, greater indulgence in alcohol and tobacco. The diet we eat is refined sugars and processed foods, and not the complex carbohydrates which was the main diet of our forefathers. All this has resulted in tremendous increase in morbidity and mortality from cardiovascular diseases.

Good health is the greatest asset we mortals can aspire to. Money cannot buy good health. All that it does is probably to mitigate our suffering. Good health is not only absence of disease but physical fitness, and physical fitness is made up of many components and attributes. A partial list would include muscular endurance, agility, cardio-respiratory efficiency, speed, balance, flexibility of the body, and tranquillity and alertness of the mind. However, it is important to remember that all people can improve their health provided they are willing to exert themselves. One has to strive for good health and unless one follows the right type of diet and proper exercises both for the mind and the body, it is not possible to achieve this goal. Yogic asanas have been planned in a masterly way by the great yogis and rishis (sages) of yore after years of observation and detailed study. The yogic practices give exercise to every system and every organ in the body, make the mind tranquil, and thus help us to keep the body healthy and the mind alert.

In the initial chapters of this book, we have dealt with the anatomy and physiology of the different systems of the body and the role of diet, alcohol, tobacco, etc., so that the reader can get a better understanding of the functions of the body and the effects produced by the different yogic practices and diet on his bodily functions and mind.

Because of numerous requests from patients and friends we have undertaken to write this book so that, even in the absence of a teacher, one can practise everyday this science of yoga in order to maintain good health. However, it is desirable, whenever possible, to get training from an expert yoga teacher.

Yogic postures will help in maintaining good health. However, people with symptoms, ailments, or disabilities should not start yogic postures without consulting their doctor. Asanas practised incorrectly may harm them, e.g. a patient of cervical spondylosis (arthritis of the neck bone) will be harmed if he practises postures which require forward bending of the neck. Those who have no ailments should carefully read the technique of each asana, its benefits and harmful effects, before starting any asana on their own.

If readers have any suggestions, they may write to us, so that we could incorporate them in the next edition.

Windsor House                                Dr. K. K. Datey
Opp. Oval Churchgate                         Dr. M. L. Gharote
Bombay 400 020                               Mr. Soli Pawri

# HEART TROUBLE?

# WHY NOT TRY YOGA.

**Is it true that heart disease is a very significant killer in society, these days?**

'Significant killer' did you say? My friend! The incidence of heart disease has more than doubled during the last fifty years.

**How intensive or extensive is the incidence?**

'Wide and deep' is the comment if that sums up the situation! Would you believe it? In the USA 54% of all deaths are due to cardiovascular disease, and every year about one million people die of this disease.

**'Cardiovascular' is a rather difficult phrase. What does it mean?**

Let's consult our good friend, the Oxford Dictionary. 'Cardio' comes from the word 'cardiac' which means 'of the heart' and 'Vascular' means 'made up of vessels or ducts for carrying blood'.

**Can we not save these people from dying if we control heart disease or, what you call 'Cardiovascular' disease ?**

How very well put! That is why, actually, research in the control and prevention of this disease has absorbed more time, money, energy and effort during the last three decades than at any time in history.

**What is the result of the research?**

You cannot expect results overnight. Though in specific areas we have come to certain conclusions, there are still some 'stubborn' areas that refuse to give us clues. The causes for over 90% of high blood pressure cases cannot be detected and out of sheer helplessness they are labelled as 'essential' hypertension.

**Isn't that funny? How can a tension, or extreme tension, or hypertension be 'essential'?**

Indeed, it is funny, but we call it 'essential' because it does occur and we have not yet found the cause, and as said before, we are helpless. Then there are cases where our arteries get hardened. This reminds me of the phrase 'hardening of attitudes' which in a sense is more dangerous than hardening of arteries.

**How come?**

Obviously, when arteries become narrow, sufficient quantity of blood is not able to flow through these blood pipes, as it were. But, when attitudes harden they prevent the flow of understanding so vital to community living. Anyway, back to hardening of arteries, the cause of this disease, is still a mystery.

**Then, has research not helped here?**

Ah, well! Research has helped us to isolate certain factors which are called the risk factors. These factors are heredity, high *cholesterol,* smoking, diabetes, and a sedentary life style.

**Most of these factors are easily understandable, but what is *cholesterol*?**

It is a crystalline substance of a fatty nature found in the brain, the nerves, the liver, the blood and the bile. It is not easily soluble. When the concentration is high in the blood it is deposited along the arterial walls, and this clogs their channels.

**But how can you at all control this disease?**

Actually efforts have been made to prevent *coronary* artery disease by control of diet and other risk factors, and by drugs.

**Any success?**

To some extent, but not entirely to our satisfaction.

What's worse, this disease does not spare even the younger age groups.

## Isn't that dreadful?

Yes, indeed, and to tell you the truth, there has been no 'breakthrough', either in curing or in prevention. But, then, it is an undisputed fact that today man is living with more stress and strain than at any time before in recorded history. Rapid advancement in science and technology has created a life-style with which man is unable to keep pace and the acquisitive standards of material advancement have set goals which are difficult to achieve.

## What has all this to do with heart disease?

My friend, haven't you heard people telling you, 'Don't take it to heart', when you feel disappointed in something or other! And so, all this has indeed a lot to do with the heart disease. You get excited over something and you are under tension. You expect your friends to understand you but they don't, and you become frustrated. You get disappointed over a case of ingratitude, you are jilted by your girl and feel as if the world is about to split into two. You get disappointed because your 'in-laws' have not come up to your expectations, — things like these do happen. Don't they?

Today with the fast pace of life, repeated changes in jobs, homes, frequent divorces and marriages, and advancement in modern technology with which man cannot keep pace, numerous tensions are created. Man is the victim of the monster he has created for himself, the monster of progress and sophistication. In this unrelenting struggle for existence he tries to keep a calm exterior but conceals a disturbed mind. Mental stress and strain is the penalty he pays for becoming more civilized. This has resulted in the phenomenal increase in psychosomatic disorders, that is, the disorders of the body caused by the disturbed mind. And so, what do these people do?

## What do people with a disturbed mind do? Do they take to drinking, smoking, become morose and gloomy, and take to permissiveness?

Yes, they do, and there begins 'the drop-out' phenomenon. Well, there is a parallel in the increase in human stress and the incidence of deaths due to heart diseases. In fact, the two appear to be interlinked. While mental stress has been regarded as a high risk factor in heart disease, there is no yardstick to measure it by, unlike other factors like high cholesterol, high blood pressure, etc., which can be determined relatively more easily.

**Then what is the real problem?**

The problem is that mental stress and strain which plays a vital role in the lives of millions today, has not received the attention it deserves. Stress is really more a psychological factor than a physical, quantifiable one. It has nevertheless become a part of human life and man has necessarily to live with it.

**Then why do doctors prescribe those horrible tranquilisers?**

Yes, horrible is the right word, but then all that is because medical science has not been able to deal with the stress element in human disease. These are all temporary measures and have no value at all. These tranquilisers only suppress the symptoms.

**I thought youngsters took to drugs because they genuinely felt 'The drug is the word'. Isn't that so?**

My friend, a drug is not a word, it is *a sentence—a life sentence!*

**Well, if drugs are not to be used, what else can be effective?**

Let us examine the problem in a simple matter-of-fact way. You will agree with me that where there is tension there is disharmony—right? Tension can be both physical and mental and therefore our approach to prevention and cure of disease should be based on the principle of *physical and mental harmony,* and it is here that we have to look back to the treasure of knowledge available to us in the annals of Yoga.

You have heard the word 'Yoga', haven't you?

**Yes, I have, but what is Yoga?**

The word 'Yoga' has been derived from the Sanskrit word 'Yuj' which means 'to join', 'to unite', 'to combine' or 'to integrate'. In this broadest sense, 'Yoga' thus means integration at three levels — *body, mind* and *soul.*

**Three levels? The soul?**

Yes, it means man must fully understand his environment and 'integrate' or become one with it. That's not enough, though. He needs to work in harmony and integrate himself with his fellow men too. But the most important thing is that he should be in harmony with his own self, his own instincts, emotions, sentiments, and ideas.

**How is that possible?**

Well, everything is possible provided you are prepared to accept this integration or what they call 'Samyama'. Haven't you heard of the phrase: an integrated personality?

**Yes, I have, but what are these instincts and emotions?**

Let me give you an example. Suppose you are in a group and you hear somebody turning to you and shouting "fire! fire!" You instinctively feel like saving yourself, don't you? You will also start saying 'fire, fire' and start running. Of course, you are scared and the members of your group, by and large, are also scared. In other words, all of you possess the common emotion of being scared. When such frightening situations happen too often you form a sort of sentiment and an idea for or against such situations. All human beings under certain conditions behave in a certain specific manner without being taught to behave that particular way. Haven't you heard of a commotion created when somebody shouts "Thief! Thief!" and when a crowd is in motion all others just instinctively follow the same crowd also shouting 'Thief! Thief!'? When man is integrated with his environment, his fellowmen and himself, he is supposed to have achieved Atma Samyam.

**What if the integration is not possible?**

Well, in that case man remains at the level of an animal, being only guided by the pull of his instincts and his wild emotions. He remains a prey to them and lives bound to the world of 'sensate culture' with no vision of a horizon which is beyond the reach of his senses. The conflict, the strain, the competition — all lead to the physical and mental disintegration of man, bringing in its trail physical or mental anxiety and uneasy emotions. This paralyses his capacity for intelligent action and to be at peace within himself.

**So, this is the philosophical basis of Yoga, is it? From where does it originate?**

Yes! That is a good question. This is indeed the philosophical basis of Yoga. You have heard of the *Bhagwat Gita*. This sacred book gives different types of Yoga. They deal with what is known as the 'Vasana' i.e. propensities or inclinations of the individuals.

**Are there many types of Yoga?**

Briefly speaking, there are three types of Yoga. The first is the *Karma Yoga*, the second is the *Bhakti Yoga*, the third *Gnyana Yoga*. Obviously, the first type, *Karma Yoga* deals with discipline, and concerns with human activity involving the control of self. *Bhakti Yoga* has something to do with the Bhakti or love and devotion to God, and *Gnyana Yoga*, as the very word suggests, has something to do with knowledge and its attainment.

**Your answers are getting more and more philosophical and rather complicated too, aren't they?**

Well, not necessarily so, if you go stage by stage, and slowly. Let's take Karma Yoga. Do you know what Karma Yoga is? It is a blend of several disciplines. Some people call it a way of life and, therefore, it could be termed Self-Control.

**But how can self-control be attained?**

Ah! that is a good question. The first thing to do is to have sense control. And how does one do that? One does it when one has a steady, governable, and controllable mind with perfect self-possession.

**It still remains difficult, doesn't it?**

Yes, it does. But our Gita tells us that one must do a thing as a social duty without expecting any reward. That means you devote yourself to the higher spirit and dedicate yourself in what you think, or say or do. The Gita believes that all human stress, strain, frustrations and disappointments are caused by self-centredness, in all our activities. Once you remove this self and do a thing without a vulgar craving for material success, you are a Karma Yogi.

**Does it mean you should not expect any reward at all?**

My friend, the reward is in the deed itself. Our object is just to do our duty, and when we concentrate on our duty devoid of all expectations, we will have a healthy body and a healthy mind.

**Do you find the same difficulty with Bhakti Yoga?**

No, it only means that if we desire to reach a goal, whatever we do must be done with love and devotion to God.

**Aren't you suggesting that 'devotion to the Lord' is a must in all our actions?**

Yes, indeed, because devotion is the central core which expresses itself into love and service to humanity and thus to God.

**And what about Gnyana Yoga?**

Gnyana Yoga is the knowledge that you acquire of being aware of yourself without delusion or illusion. This is possible only with a strict control of mind and a very high degree of mental concentration.

**This 'Gnyana' Yoga is still not understood by me, clearly. Can you elaborate it?**

I'll try. 'Gnyana' is like 'the charged power' in a steam engine which sets the engine in motion. Through 'Gnyana' we are charged with a kind of feeling of awareness or consciousness of self. Indeed, it is only when we practise this

Yoga, that we understand the meaning.

## Are these three Yogas given in the *Bhagwat Gita* mutually exclusive?

No, they are not. In fact, they are interlinked. Actually, when Karma Yoga and Bhakti Yoga are practised faithfully, they lead to 'Gnyana' Yoga, so that the first two Yogas form the cause, and 'Gnyana' Yoga the effect.

## Interesting. Anything more about these Yogas?

Yes, of course. When you do your duty without expecting any reward, you actually involve your mind in what is known as Nishkama Karma, and when the mind is involved in Bhakti you sort of surrender yourself to the Supreme Power, and for all this you need knowledge and understanding which is 'Gnyana'. So you see how beautifully the three Yogas get interlinked. In any case, what matters is the 'Bhavana'.

## Now, what exactly is this Bhavana?

'Bhavana' is an attitude of mind, and what matters more than the form is the attitude.

## Isn't all this found in Western philosophy?

Well, in a very broad sense, may be, we do talk of a proper 'attitude' towards the solution of a problem. In any case, in Hinduism or Hindu philosophy, a theory is accepted only when it is accompanied by a *practical technique*. All theoretical formulations must be given a practical application or shape.

## Do you suggest that in Hinduism there are always practical applications of a theory?

Yes. In fact, in all Hindu philosophies there are two distinct sections. Section one explains the theory and the other describes the technique or practice.

## Who pioneered this technique for practical application of Yoga?

The sage responsible for this was Patanjali, a renowned Guru. What he says is that 'Yoga Shastra' is a handy technique for applying the theory to a subjective experience which naturally will vary from individual to individual. In short, according to Patanjali, you must remember that:

(1) one must have control over one's mental faculties and (2) one should be in a position to channelise one's faculties for spiritual upliftment.

And, this spiritual upliftment means *realising one's self.*

### But how does one go about this self-realisation?

Patanjali suggests the following eight steps:

*Step No 1:* 'Control' or what he calls 'Yama'.
*Step No.2:* Culture or 'Niyama'.
*Step No.3:* Posture or 'Asana'.
*Step No.4:* Science of breathing or 'Pranayama'.
*Step No.5:* Withdrawal of senses or 'Pratyahara'.
*Step No.6:* Concentration or 'Dharana'.
*Step No.7:* Meditation or 'Dhyana'.
*Step No.8:* The final attainment or 'Samadhi'.

Thus you see this activity involves not only control so as to actually withdraw the sense-effect, but also the technique of posture, breathing, concentration, and meditation. One need not know the technical words as long as one understands what one is doing.

### I understand posture, breathing, concentration and even meditation, but I need a little more understanding of 'Yama' (Control) and 'Niyama' (Culture).

One has to understand the further stages into which these steps are sub-divided. These sub-divisions form certain codes of conduct in relation to society and the individual.

### Are these given in the religion of Hinduism?

More than religious injunctions, the code gives you helpful principles for mental and physical stability with the help of the practice of Asanas or postures, and Pranayamas or the science of breathing.

**Do the modern philosophers believe in Yoga Shastra?**

What a question ! My friend, the great scholar President of India, the late Dr. S.Radhakrishnan, described Yoga as a methodical effort to attain perfection through the control of different elements of human nature — both physical and psychical or mental. In fact, the physical body, the understanding mind and the active will are all brought under control through Yoga. It is claimed that Yoga cures the body of restlessness and frees it from its impurities. Through Yogic activities you increase your vitality, prolong youth, and promote longevity. They also tranquilise 'Chitta' or bring concentration through disciplined activity.

**But how do doctors of today react to this theory?**

To these doctors and psychologists it is a revelation. They now realise that this neglected but age-old system has exceptional values.

**How is it, there is so much misunderstanding about Yoga?**

Well, that isn't surprising. Let's enumerate some of the misunderstandings. For example,

(1) To some, Yoga means renunciation of the world — actually Yoga does not expect you to renounce the world.

(2) Some believe that to practise Yoga, one has to go to the Himalayas — Nonsense. Yoga is to to be practised by common men carrying out their daily chores of life.

(3) To some it means difficult exercises — they are really quite simple if properly understood, and carried out.

(4) Some think that Yoga is medicinal in value — yes and no; it tones up the circulatory, respiratory, digestive, and nervous systems and improves the physical and mental well-being. But, it is not only for the medicinal purposes that Yoga is practised. It has a larger bearing on the development of the whole personality.

# SKELETAL SYSTEM

**I often wonder what it is that keeps the body up—I mean, what is it that provides support to our body.**

It's the skeleton or bony system that provides a supporting framework for the body.

**Is this the only job the skeletal system does?**

No! It does many other jobs:

(a) It protects the vital organs.
(b) It provides attachement to the muscles and permits different movement of the body.

**How would you describe the skeleton?**

The human skeleton consists of two hundred and six bones and a number of cartilages. Actually the skeleton can be divided into two parts for the purposes of description, the *axial skeleton,* and the *appendicular skeleton.*

**These are difficult expressions—Will you please explain what they mean?**

Well, the part of the skeleton that forms the axis around which the body is supported is the *axial* skeleton, e.g. the backbone, the head and the chest, while the parts of the skeleton which emerge as appendages to the main skeleton form the *appendicular* skeleton.

And so, let's go into the details of these two parts.

The axial skeleton constitutes the main axis of the body and comprises:

(1) The skull (the head).
(2) The *vertebral column* or the backbone.
(3) The ribs and the breastbone.

### Does the skull mean the bones of the head?

Yes, the bones of the head as well as the bones of the face together comprise the skull. The bones of the head form what is known as the *cranium*. These bones are eight in number, they are arched and joined to provide protection to the brain. At the back of the base of the cranium there is a hole or opening called *foramen magnum* through which the spinal cord emerges.

### What about the facial bones?

They are fifteen in number and are irregular in shape and size.

### What about the backbone?

It is not one bone. It is a column of thirty three bones called *vertebrae* which you can actually feel. It is situated in the mid-line at the back of the body. Medically speaking, it is situated in the *mid-dorsal* line. It forms an axis to which all other parts of the skeleton remain attached.

### Would you say that the main job of the vertebral column is to support the body and to hold the body erect?

That is just one job — the other jobs are:

(1) to protect the delicate spinal cord and
(2) to help the movements of the trunk and the head.

### How does the vertebral column help this movement?

The vertebrae are separated from each other by discs of cartilage called intervertebral discs. Each vertebra can move slightly in relation to the next one, but these movements are restricted. It is this arrangement that makes the spine a flexible suport for the body.

## Are all the 33 vertebrae of the same structure, size or shape?

The basic plan of all the vertebrae is the same and yet there are certain differences in their structure.

Generally, we divide the spine into five regions:

Region I: The *cervical* or neck region consisting of seven vertebrae.

Region II: The *thoracic* or the chest region consisting of twelve vertebrae.

Region III: The *lumber* or the waist region consisting of five vertebrae.

Region IV & V: The *pelvic* region has the *sacrum* which is made of five sacral vertebrae fused together and the *coccyx* formed of five rudimentary vertebrae representing the vestigial tail. The sacrum lies between the two hip bones.

All vertebrae have a neural space in the middle through which the spinal cord passes.

## What about the ribs?

Well, they start from the thoracic (or chest) vertebrae and join the breastbone in the front. The breastbone is called the *sternum*. Twelve pairs of ribs form the bony thorax.

## What does the thorax with its ribs do?

They form a cage which protects the lungs, the heart, the large blood vessels, etc. The last two pairs of ribs are short and do not articulate with the sternum in front. These movements of the ribs help in the process of respiration.

## What about the appendicular skeleton?

This skeleton consists of the bones of the limbs and the girdles by which they are attached to the axial skeleton. The shoulder or the *pectoral* girdle connects the upper limbs while the pelvic girdle connects the lower limbs.

## May we know something about the shoulder girdle?

Yes, it is worth knowing that the shoulder girdle consists of the collar bone, made up of the *clavicle* in front, and the *scapula* or the shoulder blade at the back that gives us a triangular appearance. The shoulder blade is attached to the ribs and the vertebral column by means of muscles. Its upper and outer ends are attached to the arm bone (known as *humerus*). There are distinct bones for the arm, the forearm, the wrist and the fingers.

## And the other girdle?

The lower or pelvic girdle in the same manner connects the lower limbs to the vertebral column. There are two halves each of which is formed of three bones fused to each other. A deep socket at the place of fusion holds the head of the thigh bone. The lower limb consists of the thigh, the shank, the foot, and the toes—all distinct bones as in the case of the upper limb.

# MUSCULAR SYSTEM

## Why do we have muscles at all?

Well to answer that, let's exercise a little of our imagination, shall we?

(1) Can you imagine the look of a skinny-bony man without the padding of the muscles?

(2) Can you ever imagine a human being without muscles capable of moving except in ghost stories?

If our muscles were rigid and not flexible, can you imagine our human body ever having any activity at all? In fact, you use muscles for every activity. When you open and shut your eyes you use muscles. Your blood moves because of your muscles. Muscles help you to digest your food. Every kind of movement involves at least one muscle. All activities of the human body depend upon the muscles that clothe it.

## Are all the muscles of the same type?

Oh, no! If they were, it would be dreadful. In fact, the type of muscle depends upon its function.

## How many kinds of muscles are there and what are their functions?

There are three kinds of muscles:

(1) Voluntary muscles
(2) Involuntary muscles
(3) Heart muscle.

(1) *Voluntary or striated muscles:* Voluntary muscles are those that move only when you decide to move them. The cells of these muscles are longish and contain many nuclei, sometimes a hundred or more. They are also called striated muscles because when seen under a microscope, the cells look as if they have stripes or bands. These striated muscles provide force for the movement of the body. They receive their nerve supply from the voluntary nervous system. Examples of these muscles are those of your arms and legs. As a a typical example, you have seen the bulging biceps with tapering ends. These striated muscles have two ends. The

end that is attached to the most stationary portion of the skeleton is called the origin while the other end, attached to the more movable part of the skeleton, is called the insertion. The muscles are connected to the bones by what are called tendons, which are strong and flexible. Of course, they do not stretch.

(2) *Involuntary muscles:* Involuntary muscles are those that move without your control. They are also called smooth or non-striated muscles. They get their supply of nerves from the autonomic nervous system and the contraction of these muscles is almost involuntary. Examples of these muscles are those that move food through the digestive tract or alimentary canal. Their cells do not have cross stripes and each smooth muscle cell has only *one* nucleus.

## How does the cardiac or heart muscle differ from these skeletal and smooth muscles?

The heart muscle difers from the two described above, in that it is a network of *striated* muscle fibres, all interwoven. It is not the same as the smooth muscles because it has cross striations. The cardiac muscle has a rhythm—an intrinsic rhythm—and contracts rhythmically and automatically, i.e. it does not need any external stimulus. The tissue stimulation or *innervation* as it is called, in the cardiac muscle results in a wave-like contraction which passes through the entire network of the muscle fibres.

## Actually, what are the skeletal muscles composed of?

They are composed of a mixture of red and white fibres. Some of the fibres have a tinge of redness because they have large amounts of *sarcoplasm* and more muscle *haemoglobin*.

## Is there any difference in the functions of these two fibres?

Yes, muscles that have red fibres are meant for heavy and hard work and have more endurance than others. The other kind, i.e. the white muscles, are better for speed.

## How is the excessive use of the muscles possible?

The supply of capillaries to muscle tissue is quite sufficient to meet the metabolic demands of exercise.

## How do the muscles cause movement?

By contraction. For example, when you lift your arm, the big biceps muscle in your upper arm contracts and pulls the forearm upward. At the same time, the triceps muscle on the underside of your arm is relaxed. Now, the muscles cause movement in only one direction. They cannot push but can certainly pull. So, you relax the biceps to lower your arm and at the same time you contract the triceps to pull your arm back to its original position.

## Do we use the muscles the same way when lifting things?

Lifting needs more energy and so the biceps are larger and stronger muscles. That is why weight lifters, carpenters, and all those who use their arms develop large and powerful biceps.

## And what about the jaws?

The jaws? Why, you need more effort to close than to open them and that is why the muscles which close your jaws are stronger than those that open them.

## What happens to the muscles when we are at rest?

That's a good question. Even at rest, the muscles are in a state of contraction, but the contraction is just slight and is called tone. We'll talk about this a little later.

## What makes your muscles move?

It's the nerves. Nerves are connected to each muscle and receive messages. The messages are transmitted from your brain via the spinal cord or sometimes even directly from the spinal cord itself.

It's the nerves that trigger the muscles to contract or relax and, of course, in the ultimate analysis, it is your thoughts that control the action of your voluntary or skeletal muscles.

**But, what about the involuntary muscles? How are they triggered to move?**

They are sent into operation by factors over which you and I have no direct control. For example, when food is pushed onwards, it is actually done by the pressure it applies to the walls of the alimentary canal at various points. It is this pressure that causes the muscles to contract and relax. They are almost like the ripples we see in the water. Doctors call this movement *peristalsis* which keeps the food moving.

**But, what about the movement of the blood in the blood vessels?**

This too is automatic. For example, when you become hot, the walls of the blood vessels underneath the surface of the skin automatically begin to relax.

**Why?**

Because more blood is needed and so this relaxation allows more blood to enter the vessels which themselves move closer to the surface and you cool off a little.

**And when you feel cold? Does the opposite happen?**

Yes, the muscles around the blood vessels tighten, constricting their size, and reduce the amount of blood brought close to the surface, and at the same time the blood vessels themselves are pulled further below the surface.

**Where do the muscles get their strength from?**

The movement of any muscle requires energy which, as you already know, comes from the food you eat. The digested food is then carried by the blood to the muscle tissues (see digestive system). Certain foods give us more energy and that energy is stored, and because of this stored energy you can run about or do any exercise without taking food at the same time.

**What happens to our muscles when we are tired?**

When you have exhausted or finished up your energy, you get tired and your muscle cells are filled up with waste products. As you rest, the wastes are changed into carbon dioxide and water to be carried away from the muscles by the blood.

## Is it correct to say that the body movement is the work of both the muscles and the nerves?

Positively, but the point to remember here is that this body movement depends upon the combined action of the muscles and the nerves. This combined action is what is commonly known as muscular coordination.

## Can one develop this muscle coordination?

Why not? When developing muscular coordination you must first think about the movement. What you need is 'muscular skill and coordination', and you don't acquire this skill without practice. Now, do you understand why a musician practises for hours and hours. The same is true of a craftsman or even a sportsman. Indeed, to be a Don Bradman or a Sunil Gavaskar you need to practise to such an extent that coordinated movement will require a minimum of thinking and become almost automatic.

## What do you mean by 'muscular tone' of which you talked earlier?

Muscular tone determines the efficiency of a muscle.

## How is that done?

It depends upon the reaction of the nervous system to a certain stimulus. One may be at complete rest, but that does not mean the muscle has lost its tone or form.

## How does the muscle tone change?

It changes reflexly, and exercise as a rule improves the tone.

## Any cautions?

Yes, indeed, over exertion must be avoided.

**Why?**

Quite obviously they produce two types of muscular pain:

(1) Pain during and after exercise, and
(2) A localised, delayed soreness that appears in 24 to 48 hours. However, yogic postures result in static stretching which actually is very effective in removing cramps and preventng soreness.

# RESPIRATORY SYSTEM

**What is it that life needs to carry out the processes in the human body, and where does one get that from?**

Even a schoolboy knows that energy is vital to life, and the chief source of energy is food.

**How does food give energy?**

This too is very elementary. The food substances which are absorbed by the body are burnt or oxidised to yield energy. At the same time carbon dioxide is liberated along with water.

**Which is the system that does this job of oxidation and the subsequent rejection of carbon dioxide and water?**

It is the *respiratory system*, the special function of which is to provide oxygen and eliminate carbon dioxide and water which are the waste products that occur during tissue activity. Actually, there are two different types of respiration that take place in the body. These are: (i) external respiration and (ii) internal or tissue respiration.

**How do you differentiate them?**

As the word 'external' suggests, you take the oxygen from outside the body, viz. from the air. This atmospheric air is transferred to the blood and carbon dioxide is eliminated by the lungs.

**And the internal respiration takes place within the body, does it?**

Very true. The oxygen taken in by the blood is distributed to the cells, and carbon dioxide is collected from the cells.

**How does that take place?**

It is done by the process of exchange. All tissue cells are within the range of the thin-walled blood vessels known as the capillaries. The two gases, viz. oxygen and carbon dioxide, are exchanged and in this process there is a change in the colour of the blood from bright red to dusky blue.

**Is that all?**

No, one has also to remember that this exchange of gases from the air to the blood, from the blood to the tissues, and from the tissues back to the blood is done by the process of diffusion. Further, for the exchange of gases in the lungs a large amount of blood is needed as the blood has to be exposed to the atmospheric air.

**What do the lungs look like?**

They are spongy pink-coloured organs. We say lungs because they are two. They are extremely thin-walled and their surface has a large area, but it is accommodated in a small space.

**How is that done?**

They are folded into small sacks, which the doctors call *alveoli*. These alveoli are lined by a single layer of cells. The lungs also have a dense and close network of thin-walled blood vessels called capillaries.

**Why should there be so many and why should they be thin-walled?**

Don't forget, the gases are to be exchanged and the thin walls of alveoli and capillaries facilitate that instantaneously. For this an extensive net-work is necessary because the lungs are a factory that purify blood through this exchange. What actually happens in this factory is that the lungs expand and compress, as can be easily felt by the movements like the heaving of the chest, and this results in the air being inhaled and exhaled.

**We take in air through our nose and at times through the mouth, don't we?**

We do so, but there is a pipe that connects our nose and mouth to the lungs and this is commonly known as the wind pipe which the doctors call the *trachea*.

**Now, let's talk of this wind pipe a little more, shall we?**

The nose leads to what are known as the *pharynx* and the *larynx,* and from there to the trachea. The trachea (the wind pipe) divides into two branches known as the *bronchi,* and these enter into the lungs. These bronchi further divide into smaller branches known as *bronchioles,* which still further sub-divide to form the terminal bronchiole which leads into the alveoli or the air sacs.

**How do they maintain their tubular form so that they don't collapse?**

That is a sensible question. You see, there are rings made of cartilage, which keeps the trachea and the bronchi open. This is necessary, particularly when the pressure is low, lest the tubes get closed.

**What about the inside of the trachea and the bronchi?**

These respiratory passages are covered with numerous hair medically known as *cilia,* which constantly move to and fro.

**Why should they do that?**

Well, with the polluted air that we breathe in, it is necessary to have some device which can trap dust particles and bacteria. Besides, there is the mucus to help the cilia to trap these dust particles.

**Where do these impurities go?**

These impurities are mopped up and swept into other organs known as the larynx and the *oesophagus,* from where you either swallow them or spit them out .

**How are these delicate and spongy lungs protected?**

They are in the closed chest cavity known as the *thorax.* This cavity, as you can feel yourself, is made of ribs, twelve on either side. They are connected to the spine or the vertebral column behind and to the breast bone (or *sternum*) in front.

## What about the bottom of this cavity?

The bottom is just a muscular sheet which naturally is also the top of the abdominal cavity below. This is called the *diaphragm*.

## How does the chest cavity alter its shape and size?

It is the muscles that change the size and shape of the thoracic or chest cavity. But mind you, within this cavity the lungs also expand and contract, and yet the two movements are synchronised to permit unhindered breathing.

## But how does this take place?

Each lung is covered by a *serous membrane* which is in the form of a sac, termed the *pleura*. The inner part of this serous membrane covers the surface of the lungs, while the outer part lines the inner surface of the corresponding part of the chest wall. The two layers are continuous with each other, and the potential space between them is known as the pleural cavity. In between the two layers is a sort of lubricating fluid, which facilitates the easy gliding movement.

## But how does breathing itself take place?

The muscles of the thorax (chest) contract and relax bringing about the movement of the diaphragm and chest wall and this results in air being inhaled and exhaled. The process of respiration can be divided into two phases: (1) inspiration and (2) expiration.

When respiration takes place there are two movements. The first is breathing in and for that:

(1) The muscles of the diaphragm contract and make it flat. (In the relaxed state the diaphragm is dome-shaped).

(2) The abdominal organs are pushed down as it were and the volume of the chest cavity increases.

(3) Now the muscles between the ribs contract and make the ribs move upward and outward.

(4) The volume of the thoracic cavity having increased, the lungs find room to expand, and the atmospheric air rushes in. The inspiration is over.

**What is next?**

That's simple. Now breathing out or expiration begins.
How?

1. The muscles of the diaphragm relax.
2. The muscles between the ribs, too, relax.
3. The diaphragm is pushed back into its dome-shape.
4. The ribs move down.
5. The lungs return to their original volume; and
6. The air is pushed out.

A point to be remembered here is that in quiet breathing
the major role in respiration is played by the diaphragm.

# NERVOUS SYSTEM

## What is it that regulates the various systems in the body?

Strange as it may seem, it's a special system that regulates all other systems to meet the bodily requirements.

## When does it function?

All the time, and under both normal and abnormal conditions which include, of course, stress and strain.

## Where does it function?

Within the body, of course, at what they call nerve-centres which control all the movements of the body whether autonomic or otherwise.

The part of the nervous system that helps in autonomic or sub-conscious regulation is called the *autonomic nervous system;* while the part which controls body musculature and also influences the autonomic nervous system is called the *somatic system.*

## What are the different parts of this nervous system?

They are—the brain, the spinal cord and, of course, the nerves. They are like the different sections of a telegraphic system.

## Why do you say 'telegraphic'?

Because it deals with 'messages' as the telegraph system does. The nervous system of the body gets messages from various parts of the body through innumerable nerve cells known as *receptors.*

## 'Receptors'—because they receive messages?

Yes. The receptors then do their job by sending the

messages to the nerve centres through special nerves called the sensory nerves.

### What do the nerve centres do then?

Well, they interpret the messages and send orders through another set of nerves called the motor nerves. This is done through a pathway known as the *reflex arc,* and the action which takes place in response to a certain stimulus is called a reflex action.

### Can you please clarify all this?

Yes, why not? Take this example: Suppose you touch something very hot; what happens? Your hand gets withdrawn instantaneously, doesn't it?

### Why, yes. Please tell me something more about it.

For the sake of convenience, the nervous system may be divided into two sections, the *central* nervous system and the *peripheral* nervous system.

The first system—the central one, consists of the brain and the spinal cord both of which are well protected by bony structures. Let's first talk about the brain.

(1)  When we say 'brain', we actually mean all its parts, viz., the *cerebrum,* the *cerebellum* and the brain-stem which itself is made up of the *medulla* and the *pons.*

(2)  The brain including the brain-stem is covered by a protective membrane called the *meninges.*

(3)  The cerebrum is the largest part of the brain.

### How large?

It's about ⅔rd of the whole brain. It consists of two hemispheres—two cerebral halves—the right and the left.

### Are they two separate halves?

The answer is 'yes' and 'no'. They are separate but are connected below by a bundle of nerve fibres and their medical name is *'Corpus Callosum'*. One more piece of information about the cerebrum is that its outer region consists of grey matter which too has a medical name — *'Cerebral Cortex'*. The cortex has an increased surface area and like the 'air sacs' of the lungs, a vast area is accommodated in a small space by a pattern of convolutions or folds.

### Is it true of other animal cortices too?

Yes, the cortices of animal brains also have convolutions, but since man's brain is well developed, it has more convolutions.

### Oh, I see! That's why we say an intelligent man has more grey matter—isn't it?

Yes, in a way. But to come back to the cortex, what lies below is the white matter, which actually is a bundle of nerve fibres.

### To what are the fibres connected?

Some of them connect the different parts of the cerebrum itself, while others connect the cerebrum to the other parts of the brain. In the cerebral hemispheres there are cavities called *ventricles* which contain the *cerebrospinal fluid*.

### All this is too technical, but what is the actual function of the cerebrum?

The cerebrum apart from being the centre of motor and sensory control is also the seat of consciousness, intelligence, memory, imagination, and even reasoning. One side of the cerebral hemisphere controls the activities of the opposite side of the body. Of course, for every specific activity there is a specific area, and as you perhaps know, there are different centres for hearing, sight, taste, speech, etc., etc.

**Does that mean that damage to a particular area of the brain affects a particular activity?**

Yes, and now let's talk of what is below and behind the cerebrum, viz. the cerebellum. It has a peculiar shape—a middle portion and two lobes on the sides. The grey matter and the white matter are also there on the outer and inner side respectively.

**What does the cerebellum do?**

When you walk, run or dance, your muscles are under the control of this part of the brain. In fact, the cerebellum is the balancing agent of your body.

**What about the third part of the brain—the stem?**

I was about to come to that, for the stem contains a portion of both the parts we have talked about, the cerebrum and the cerebellum. As a matter of fact, it has a third part too, the spinal cord. Right in the middle of the brain stem there is a nerwork of nerve cells and nerve fibres which group into the cortex and down into the spinal cord.

**What about the functions of the brain-stem?**

The brain-stem contains many important nerve centres, viz.

(i)     The respiratory centre,
(ii)    The cardiac centre or the centre pertaining to the heart,
(iii)   The vasomotor centre or the centre pertaining to the blood vessels, and
(iv)    The salivary or deglutition centre.

**What is the word 'deglutition'?**

'Deglutition' means 'swallowing'. And now to the spinal cord, the importance of which you cannot even imagine.

**The spinal cord is in the backbone, isn't it?**

So it is. It is actually the long 'tail' as if it were a continuation of the brain and is a tubular structure. The vertebral column has the neural canal, through which the spinal cord passes. It starts from the brain and goes right upto the end of the tail.

**What about the grey matter? Does it have this matter?**

Of course, it has both the grey matter and the white matter but with this difference that, in the cerebrum and the cerebellum, the grey matter is on the outside and the white inside, but in the spinal cord it is in the *reverse* — it is the *white* matter which is on the outside, while the *grey* matter is on the inside.

**But if the whole spinal cord is enclosed within the vertebral column, how can the nerves go out?**

That's a sensible question. The vertebral column is not one rigid bone, it is made of separate bone pieces known as vertebrae. Between the vertebrae there is space and through these spaces between the vertebrae shoot out nerves like the branches shooting out on the two sides of the stem of a leaf or plant. The nerves emerge and travel to different parts of the body.

**And what are the functions of the spinal cord?**

Its functions are twofold:

(1) It conducts messages or impulses to and from the brain, and
(2) It acts as a reflex centre.

And now we go on to the *peripheral system*.

**What's that?**

We did talk about it earlier — didn't we?

Any way, you'll understand it as we go along. This nervous system is divided into — (i) the cranial and the spinal nerves and (ii) the autonomic nerves.

# AUTONOMIC NERVOUS SYSTEM AND YOGA PRACTICES

**What do you mean by the term autonomic nervous system?**

The ANS (as the autonomic nervous system is called) is that part of the nervous system which regulates bodily functions other than those of free volition, i.e. voluntary movements and bodily sensations.

**Does this system have any specific nerves?**

Yes, it has two types of nerves:

(a) Sympathetic nerves
(b) Parasympathetic nerves

**But is it not true that most of the organs receive nerve supply from both the sets?**

Yes, you are right. Both the sets supply the nerves which regulate the functions of these organs.

**Then what is so special about the ANS?**

The ANS is also intimately connected with the *endocrine* system, and the *hypothalamus*.

**I don't understand either 'Endocrine' or 'Hypothalamus'?**

I quite appreciate your difficulty. Endocrine glands are ductless glands and hypothalamus is the highest centre for both endocrine system and ANS.

**But what are the functions of the two types of nerves, the sympathetic and the parasympathetic?**

Actually the two subdivisions have opposite effects: While the sympathetic system stimulates the organ, the parasympathetic 'depresses' it, and vice versa.

**Can you give an example?**

I can give you a number of examples. For instance:

(1) If the pupil of the eye is dilated by the sympathetic activity, the parasympathetic constricts it.
(2) If the sympathetic activity raises the blood pressure, the parasympathetic lowers it.
(3) If the sympathetic inhibits the activity of the stomach and the intestine, the parasympathetic stimulates it.
(4) If the sympathetic increases the heart rate, the parasympathetic slows it down.

## But what exactly is the parasympathetic concerned with?

In general, we may say that the parasympathetic is concerned with functions serving the *regeneration* of the organs while the sympathetic is concerned with the job of mobilising the latent reserves of the organs, when special efforts are needed.

## All this denotes maintaining a certain type of balance, doesn't it?

That's right. Usually there is a very fine regulatory balance between the two activities in the organism.

## Is this balance ever disturbed?

Of course, it is. Under certain conditions the balance is disturbed.

## Who discovered this balance?

A psychologist named Wenger calls it the 'autonomic balance of an individual'. If the two are not well-balanced the activity of the one dominates over the other, and this results in autonomic imbalance.

## What can help if the balance is upset?

The discipline of yoga can help. Serious yoga students are known to have the ability to relax voluntarily because yogic practices do modify the autonomic functions in general by increasing the parasympathetic function to the betterment of the individual.

# ENDOCRINE SYSTEM

**Isn't it strange that some of us are very tall, some are dwarfish, some have long noses like that of Cyrano de Bergerac, or bulbous ones like Pinnochio's or some have jumbo ears and some have very small ones. Is there no regular pattern of growth for us?**

That is a very sensible and intelligent question. The answer to that is: Yes, every one has his or her pattern of growth and that growth is controlled by a system composed of a number of small special glands located in various parts of the body.

**But, I thought it's the nerves that control the body's activities, don't they?**

Yes, they do, but their functions are quite distinct and different. Nerves are connected to one another, and messages are sent along them as along telegraphic wires, but the system which controls our growth pattern helps to control body activities in a manner different from that of the nervous system.

**What is the difference and why?**

Nerves govern immediate and fast moving actions such as muscle movements, and have a temporary effect on the body. But this new system—

**Sorry for the interruption, but what do you call this system?**

It is called the *'Endocrine System'*. Actually, it is a sort of chemical control. The endocrine glands control activities that are generally slower but have a longer or permanent effect on the body.

**How is that done? Is the control through wires or some sort of nerves?**

No, the control by the glands is indirect—they release special chemicals into the blood.

**What do you call these special chemicals?**

They are called *hormones* and it is these hormones that determine the rate and type of our growth and development.

It is these hormones that control our behaviour and have a lot to do with the shaping of our personality.

**Which and where are these glands?**

The most important one, — the master gland as it were — is a very small gland (*pituitary*) located at the base of the brain. In fact, a part of the gland is attached to the brain by a narrow stalk through which it continues with the brain. It has two lobes: (i) *anterior lobe,* (ii) *posterior lobe*.

**What is the function of this gland?**

As I told you, it produces what we call hormones.

**Can you tell us something more about these hormones?**

The anterior lobe secretes the growth hormone, the milk-producing hormone, the hormone influencing sugar and fat metabolism, and the hormones influencing other glands.

**What are those other glands?**

They are the *thyroid,* the *adrenals,* the *parathyroids,* and the *sex glands*. As stated above, one of the hormones of the anterior pituitary is the growth hormone which determines our growth pattern. Too much of this produces giants.

**And I suppose too little of it, dwarfs—right?**

Right, indeed. The abnormal size of ears, nose, feet, hands, etc. are all results of this hormone playing havoc with the body.

**What does the posterior lobe of the pituitary control?**

The posterior lobe controls the amount of water stored in the body and ultimately affects blood pressure.

### What about the other glands—the thyroid gland, for instance?

This is located in the neck just above the voice box, which as you know is called the *larynx*.

### What is the function of the thyroid gland?

The function of this gland is to set the pace as it were for the control of the basic processes of the body through its hormone. That is why it is called the pace setter. It specially affects the growth pattern.

### In what way?

Children, for example, with too little of this hormone (*hypothyroidism*) become mentally and physically retarded. In adults, its deficiency causes fattiness, weakness, nervousness, and mental sluggishness.

### Is there no cure for this?

Of course there is—by giving thyroid hormone as a replacement therapy to patients of hypothyroidism.

### Is there a special name for this hormone?

Yes, indeed, it is called *thyroxine*.

### What happens when excess of this hormone (thyroxine) is secreted?

It causes increase in pulse rate, tremors, prominent eyes, swelling in neck, palpitation and loss of weight.

### How do we control this condition?

Formerly surgical removal of the gland was the remedy, but, today most of the patients can be controlled with medical treatment.

### Is the thyroid gland separate by itself?

No, behind it are the glands we call the parathyroids which are four in number.

**You have used the word Parathyroids before. What does it mean?**

These are four small yellowish pea-sized glands.

**But, what is the function of the parathyroids?**

Their function is to control the calcium metabolism.

**Are there any other glands?**

Yes, of course. At the top of each kidney is a pyramid-shaped gland known as the *adrenal gland*. Its inner portion is called the *medulla* while the outer layer is known as the *cortex*.

**What are its functions?**

The medulla produces a hormone known as *adrenaline* which is also called the emergency hormone. It causes the liver to release more sugar into the blood.

**Why is it called emergency hormone?**

If you have seen a bloody fight between two boxers, who with their faces smeared with blood, fight tenaciously on, you will realise that there is something in them that keeps them going. And that something is the emergency adrenaline which helps them make herculean or superhuman efforts, to carry their fight on with bleeding faces.

**What about the cortex?**

It is the outer layer of the adrenal gland which yields several other hormones.

**And what do these hormones do?**

They have a variety of functions to perform! Here are some —

(1)  They control the sugar level in the body.

(2)  They influence the salt and water excretion from the kidneys

(3)  They also govern the secondary sexual characteristics.

## What do you mean by secondary sexual characteristics?

These are the growth of the beard in the case of males and of the breasts in the case of females!

## Where else do we find these endocrine glands?

Well within the pancreas, we find groups of endocrine cells. These cells secrete a special hormone known as insulin.

## What is the use of this insulin?

It is essential for proper utilisation of sugar in the body. Without this hormone the body cells do not use the sugar in the blood stream, and this causes the disease known as 'Diabetes'.

## What is the effect of Yoga on the different endocrine glands?

The yogic postures and breathing exercises are so well planned that they influence all the endocrine glands and bring all the bodily functions to the optimum level. This helps to correct the dysfunctions of the organs. If one is over-weight, he loses weight; if one is underweight, he gains in weight. The effects of these postures and breathing exercises have been discussed in the individual chapters.

# CARDIOVASCULAR SYSTEM

## What does this big word mean?

I have told you earlier that the word 'cardio' comes from 'cardiac' which means 'pertaining to the heart' and 'vascular' stands for the vessels that carry blood.

## What are the parts of this system? What do they do?

The blood, the blood vessels, and the heart are the main parts of this system. Actually, the blood vessels form a communicating system with all the living parts of the body. As you know, the heart has a pumping action which keeps the blood in circulation and helps in the distribution of the blood to all the parts of the body through the blood vessels.

## How is that done?

Before we go to that question, let's remember a few facts.

(1) Blood in a blood vessel always flows in the same direction.
(2) It passes repeatedly through the heart.
(3) The blood vessels are of three types:
   (a) The arteries.
   (b) The capillaries, and
   (c) The veins.

## Must we know all these details?

Yes, otherwise you will not understand the system. After all, each type of blood vessel has its own function. Let's take stock of these blood vessels.

(1) The first is the *artery*. It carries blood away from the heart, i.e. from the heart to the limbs and other organs of the body.
(2) Arteries are wide, thick-walled, muscular, and elastic. If you have been to a city reservoir of water you must have noticed that the pipes that leave the reservoir are usually thick, wide, and strong, since they carry a large amount of water and these then taper down to narrower pipe lines before they reach the house tap. Much the same way these arteries divide into smaller vessels.

### Is there any special name for these smaller vessels?

Yes, these smaller vessels are called *arterioles* which further divide into still smaller vessels called *capillaries*.

### What is the function of the capillaries?

These capillaries also carry blood, but they are responsible for carrying the blood to every single cell in the body. Unlike those of the arteries or arterioles, the walls of the capillaries are very thin and permeable.

### How does that help?

Because they are thin and permeable, they allow the gases (oxygen and carbon dioxide), water and the dissolved substance in the blood to diffuse into and out of the tissues.

### And then?

Then eventually the capillaries once again unite and form larger and larger vessels called the *veins*.

### What do these veins do?

Their job is to return the impure blood to the heart. So you see, pure blood starts from the heart and the impure blood *goes back* to the heart.

### How about telling us something about the heart itself?

It's a muscular pump, as it were. Here are some of the facts:

(1) Size     — That of the fist of the individual
(2) Weight   — 300 gms approx. in a male adult and about 50gms less in a female.
(3) Muscles  — It is made of special muscles—not ordinary muscles. Why? Because the incessant beating of the heart would exhaust ordinary muscles. It is tough and resilient, recuperates rapidly, and is none the worse for its wear and tear. In other words, it is inexhaustible.

### What is the name of this special kind of muscle?

It is called the *myocardium*, and the membrane that covers this muscle on the outside is called the *pericardium;* while the lining inside is called the *endocardium*.

### Does it mean that the myocardium is wrapped up and sandwiched between the pericardium on the outer side and the endocardium on the inside?

Yes, you could say that. Now let's have a peep inside the heart. We see four chambers. The two thin-walled chambers are the *atria or auricles* and the two thicker wall-ed, the *ventricles*. These four chambers are arranged into two compartments, the right and the left. The right compartment has the right atrium above and the right ventricle below. Similarly, the left compartment has the left atrium above and the left ventricle below. As there has to be a door to let the blood flow from the upper to the lower chambers, there are 'one-way valves' which allow the blood to flow only in one direction, i.e. from the atria to the ventricles. The valve between the right atrium and the right ventricle is the *tricuspid valve,* and the valve guarding the opening between the left atrium and the left ventricle is called *mitral valve*. The right and the left compartments are separated by a wall, and there is no direct communication between the right and the left sides. The two atria and the two ventricles are separated by two different *septa* or partitions.

### Why are the atria thin-walled and the ventricles thick-walled?

The atria are thin-walled because they receive the blood from the veins and merely push it down to the lower chambers, i.e. the ventricles. No great effort is required for this and so they are thin. On the other hand, the ventrilcles have to pump and push the blood out into the blood vessels (pipes) with every beat of the heart. Since they have to do a strenuous job, they are thick-walled.

### But what is it that pushes the blood out?

It is the contraction of the heart which provides most of the force required to keep the blood moving.

## What happens when the heart pushes the blood out?

That's the story of the journey of the blood, otherwise known as circulation.

## But what starts it all?

The stimulation for the contraction originates in the heart itself. The action of the heart in pumping the blood starts a cyclic pattern which we will try to follow step by step.

*First step* : The great veins, i.e., the *superior vena cava* and the *inferior vena cava* empty the deoxygenated blood into the right atrium.

*Second step* : The right atrium contracts and pumps the blood into the right ventricle through the tricuspid valve.

*Third step* : In turn, the right ventricle contracts and pumps the blood into the lungs for oxygenation.

This is called the *pulmonary circuit*.

(a) The oxygenated blood from the lungs enters the left atrium.

(b) The left atrium contracts and pumps the blood into the left ventricle.

(c) In turn, the left ventricle contracts and pumps the blood into the aorta from where it flows to all parts of the body through the arteries and the capillary network. The oxygen from the blood is taken up by the cells of the body and deoxygenated blood is returned to the right atrium through the great veins.

This constitutes the *systemic circuit*.

And this cycle continues. Incidentally, at first the two atria contract almost simultaneously followed by the contraction of the ventricles.

## How often does this happen?

It's amazing, but within just one minute, the heart beats about 70 to 75 times.

**What about the impure blood? Does it not accumulate within the body?**

Don't forget, nature has taken care of that, too. No, the impure blood doesn't get accumulated. It gets oxygenated in the lungs.

**How does the blood flow in the two systems?**

The pulmonary circuit is a short one in as much as the blood goes from the right atrium to the right ventricle, the pulmonary artery, and the network of capillaries in the lungs where the blood gets oxygenated, i.e. purified, and then goes to the pulmonary vein and from there to the left atrium.

The other circuit known as the systemic circuit involves the left atrium, the left ventricle, the *aorta* or the biggest artery, its branches, the capillary network in the various parts of the body, the big veins known as the Superior Vena Cava and the Inferior Vena Cava—and then the right atrium, the right ventricles from where the other circuit begins again. You must have realised that this circuit is concerned with the job of circulating blood throughout the body except, of course, in the lungs where the other circuit, i.e. the pulmonary one, works.

**But what does blood do actually as it flows through the body?**

It provides nutrients and oxygen to the tissues and collects the waste products from them.

# DIGESTIVE SYSTEM

**Why does the body need food at all?**

The body needs food for three main purposes:

(1) For producing energy to do the daily work.

(2) For creating new cells and tissues in order to promote growth, and

(3) For renewing the worn-out cells and tissues.

**But what are the foods the body needs?**

The body needs two sets of food. The first set includes proteins, fats, and carbohydrates, while the second set includes minerals, vitamins, and water. You must remember that the first group, viz.proteins, fats and carbohydrates have to be converted into simple chemcial substances in order to be absorbed or digested, but the second group, i.e., the minerals, vitamins, and water, do not need any change and can be absorbed by the body as such. In fact, what we call digestion really means the conversion of complex organic material into simple substances which would be helpful and suitable for absorption by the body. The system that is specially resposible for the process of absorption, conversion, and digestion is called the *'digestive system'*.

**Where does the process take place?**

It takes place in what we call the alimentary canal (tract).

**Where and what is this canal?**

It begins at the mouth, is about eight metres long, and ends at the anus.

**Eight metres, i.e. 26 ft. long, in a man five to six feet tall?**

Yes, but it is coiled up in the abdominal cavity.
To understand it properly let us divide it into six convenient parts:

Part 1.    Mouth          Part 4.    Stomach
Part 2.    Pharynx        Part 5.    Small intestine
Part 3.    Oesophagus     Part 6.    Large intestine.

Each of these parts has different functions to perform.

But, before we discuss these functions, let us keep in mind the fact that the process of digestion in these parts takes place with the help of certain organs.

**And which are they?**

They are—(1) The salivary glands
         (2) The liver, and
         (3) The pancreas.

The salivary glands and the other two organs secrete certain juices as the food passes through the alimentary canal. And now, back to the different parts of the canal.

*Part 1. The mouth:* The mouth receives the food, and with the help of the teeth and the tongue, grinds it into small fragments. The saliva from the salivary glands pours in and the food so mixed up forms into what is called a *bolus.*

*Part 2. The pharynx:* The masticated food has to be swallowed and this is done with the help of the pharynx.

*Part 3. The oesophagus:* This is a ten-inch long muscular tube that receives the bolus swallowed with the help of the pharynx.

The walls of this tube contract and relax to push the food down to the stomach, i.e. part 4.

**How does the food go down the tube during and after a meal even when we lie flat?**

That is an intelligent question. It would be wrong to suppose that the food goes down because of the action of gravity. The walls of the oesophagus have circular and also longitudinal (lengthwise) muscle fibres. By the alternate contraction and relaxation of these muscles, the bolus is pushed onwards into the stomach, i.e. part 4.

**The stomach?**

Yes, the stomach is a pouch, a reservoir of food. It is here that partial digestion takes place. Now we shall continue with the journey of our morsel. The stomach with the help of its own muscles, pushes the food, partially digested by the *gastric juices*, into the small intestine.

**This is part 5, isn't it?**

Right, so it is, and here in Part 5 (the small intestine), the rest of the digestion takes place.

**And what about part 6 or the large intestine?**

Well, that's almost the end of the journey. The remaining portion is passed into the large intestine which absorbs most of the water and finally discards the waste or the residue as faeces which we excrete in the toilet.

**How does the digestion take place?**

For this we begin with the mouth, i.e. back to Part 1. We saw earlier that the food is first mixed with the saliva, a digestive juice. There are actually *three pairs* of salivary glands. These glands have ducts which open in the mouth and thus pour the saliva.

**What is this saliva?**

The saliva contains an enzyme called *ptyalin* which acts on cooked starch and turns it into *maltose*. Saliva also contains a substance called *mucin* which acts like a lubricant. It lubricates the food and makes the particles adhere to one another to form bolus. There is a centre in the brain which controls the secretion of saliva. The moment we see food we are fond of, or even smell it, the centre is stimulated and secretion begins.

**Oh, I see! Is that why we say 'my mouth begins to water'?**

That's correct! Yes, we do say that. Why! sometimes when we are hungry even the thought of food excites this centre and the salivary glands begin to secrete. Anyway, what we must remember here is that at stage 1 the starch of the food becomes maltose. The next stage of digestion i.e. stage 2 is in the stomach.

## What happens in the stomach?

The *pyloric end* (the distal end) closes and the food remains in the stomach for a certain period before it is pushed into the small intestine. The lining of the stomach has glands which secrete the gastric juice. It is a continuous secretion, but it increases with meals.

## What does this gastric juice contain?

It contains hydrochloric acid as well as two other enzymes namely *pepsin* and *renin*. Hydrochloric acid provides the right medium or pH for the enzymes pepsin and renin to act.

## What does pepsin do?   It breaks up protein into peptides.

## And renin?      Renin clots the milk protein.

## Has the stomach any role?

The stomach has what they call a peristaltic movement which churns the food, mixing it up with the gastric juice and converting it into a creamy fluid called *chyme*.

## How long does food remain in the stomach, and what happens?

It depends—mainly on the type of food present in it. It varies from a few minutes to an hour or sometimes even three hours (average about two hours).

In the mouth, the starch becomes maltose, and in the stomach, the proteins are broken into peptides and the food changes into *chyme*.

## What happens next?

Well, the journey isn't over, the chyme has to move on, and so it does and the journey is a pretty long one, as long as twenty feet (six metres).

**Twenty feet?**

Yes, but the path again can be divided into three parts—the *duodenum*, the *jejunum*, and the *ileum*.

**What happens then?**

A special juice—the bile formed in the liver—flows through the bile duct into the duodenum. The bile, with the help of another juice, the pancreatic juice (which, as the name suggests, comes from the pancreas) breaks up proteins into peptones, and peptides into amino acids and starch (cooked and even uncooked) into maltose.

**What about fats?**

The bile salts help to activate certain enzymes and they break up fats into fatty acids and *glycerol*.

**And all this happens in the small intestine?**

Yes, even the small intestine has special glands which secrete/produce certain enzymes. These enzymes complete the process of digestion. And the place where most of the ab sorption takes place is the *ileum*.

**Does it mean that everything one eats gets absorbed completely?**

No, there is always some unabsorbed food which then moves on to the large intestine.

**Does the large intestine have its own glands?**

Yes, but the large intestine has only one secretion, *mucin*, which lubricates the unabsorbed residual food in order ot facilitate its passage out through the rectum. The large intestine or the *colon* absorbs water and the semi solid faeces are passed into the rectum and are finally excreted through the anus.

**How does the food move on?**

The same way as it did in the stomach—the peristaltic movement.

# EXCRETORY SYSTEM

**We have the urge to go to the toilet every day just as we feel hungry every day—why does this happen?**

We eat to build up our body, but we go to the toilet to throw out wastes. Doctors use the term *'metabolic' process* for this.

**What does that mean?**

It is a term that describes the process of tissue building on the one hand, and cell distruction on the other. The first process has a special name called *anabolism*. The cell-breaking, or rather, the breaking down of the tissues *(catabolism)* produces what we in medical language call *toxic metabolites*.

**Toxic? What does that mean?**

Toxic means poisonous—and, therefore, our body has a system by which these poisons are thrown out.

**Yes, we have learnt that the function of the blood is not only to provide oxygen, but also to take away carbon dioxide and thus blood is a part of this elimination system, isn't it?**

Yes, you could put it that way. Wastes of several kinds are eliminated by the body.

**What organs perform this elimination work?**

There are several organs which do this work, the lungs, the kidneys and the skin.
*Carbon dioxide* is released from the blood and the lungs throw it out when you exhale.

**Do the lungs throw out only carbon dioxide?**

No, besides carbon dioxide, they throw out water to some extent and in disease the lungs throw out many other products which are toxic. Do you know that alcohol is the only substance thrown out by the lungs of a healthy person?

**Is that why we can easily find out whether a man has had a 'drink' or not?**

Yes, indeed the lungs throw out alcohol when the person exhales and this is used for detecting the presence of alcohol with a 'Breath Analyser'.

This is a simple test and is used by the police in the .Western countries for detecting whether a car driver has imbibed alcohol.

**What about the stuff we eat? Why, once I heard that my little baby cousin swallowed a little bead but when given a castor oil purge, the bead was in his stool! How come?**

That's because the solid (bead) was indigestible. In fact, solid indigestible materials are thrown out of the body, all through the food tract and the rectum as stools.

**But how is it that our stools have colour?**

The bile pigment is formed in the liver due to breakdown of the haemoglobin of the worn out red cells which is excreted in the faeces and this gives it the characteristic colour.

**What about the urine we pass?**

Urine is a liquid waste which is filtered off from the blood and contains dissolved salts.

**How is that done?**

It is done in our body's filtration plant known as the kidneys.

**Yes, I have heard about the kidneys. They are supposed to be two, isn't that correct?**

That's right. The kidneys are two in number, having the shape of beans.

**How large are they?**

They are the size of a small fist.

**Where exactly are they placed in the body?**

They are located in the abdominal cavity at the back, one on each side of the spinal cord at the level of the 12th thoracic and the upper three lumbar vertebrae.

**What is inside them?**

The kidney is a complicated thing.
(1) It has an outer layer called the *cortex*.
(2) It also has an inner layer—they call it the *medulla*.

**What are these layers made of?**

Each layer is made of small arteries, veins and capillaries, those very, very tiny tubes, thousands of them.

**Thousands of them, really?**

Yes, it's a miracle. There are so many of these tiny tubes, that if one were to place them end to end, they would cover a distance of about 60 kilometres!

**Unbelievable! But eventually where do these tubes end in?**

They eventually connect with a large tube called the ureter, which empties in a sac-like elastic organ (bladder) that holds the urine till you feel like passing it out.

**How is this carried out in the kidney?**

Like all other organs, each kidney has a large artery which brings blood into it, and an equally large vein which carries the deoxidated blood away. As in the case of the lungs, this artery divides into smaller blood vessels called arterioles and capillaries that finally end up in what is technically called the *glomerulus* which is held in a capsule.

**How many such capsules are there?**

How many, did you say? At least a million in each of these kidneys! Actually these are mazes, and as the blood passes through them it becomes purified, in the sense that it is filtered of many of its poisonous wastes.

**Would you then say that the main function of the kidneys is to filter out injurious and unwanted materials from the blood?**

Yes, indeed, urea is what it mainly filters out. Actually, urea is converted into ammonia. In fact, in doing this it brings about a balance between the acid and the alkaline bases in the body.

**How much urine does one pass normally?**

About 1.5 litres in 24 hours, depending upon the amount of water or liquid intake, sweating, etc.

**Urine may be of different colours, is it not so?**

Yes, and thank God for it. The pigment in the urine gives it the straw yellow colour. Variation in the physical and chemical compositions of urine help us to find out the diseases of the kidney, the liver, the bladder etc.

**How are the diseases indicated?**

(1) Some pass more urine.
(2) Some have difficulty in passing it.
(3) Some pass blood in urine.
(4) Some complain of backache.

For example, if one passes a large amount of urine and does it frequently, doctors may suspect diabetes. On the other hand, if urine is passed in small amounts and has albumin in it, it indicates damage to the kidneys.

**What about the perspiration? Is it also a waste and why is it that our perspiration tastes saltish?**

Our perspiration is a waste and it is salty because it is water and salt. We excrete salt and water as sweat through our skin.

**So, the skin too is a member of the excretory system, is it?**

Indeed it is, but it does many things besides. In fact, it is called the 'Jack of all trades'.

(1) It covers and protects the entire outer surface of our body. In fact, it is a tight fitting sack that holds the body.

(2) Every square centimetre of the skin contains:
(a) several sweat glands,
(b) dozens of oil glands,
(c) three feet of tiny capillaries carrying blood to and fro from the skin,
(d) about 12 feet of nerves which sense heat, cold, touch, pressure and pain, and of course, thousands of skin cells.

**How can one see the sweat glands?**

You cannot see the glands, but with the help of a magnifying glass you can see the openings of these glands. They look like small pits.

**But why do we sweat?**

Why! It's the body's temperature regulator. The body normally loses heat in three ways.
—Radiation
—Conduction
—Evaporation
In hot weather we sweat more, and this prevents the body temperature from rising. Similary, in cold weather perspiration is very, very little, which helps to maintain the body temperature and prevents it from going down.

# YOGIC EXERCISES (POSTURES)
# AND
# PHYSICAL EXERCISES

**Why do you call yogic exercises postures? Are they not exercises?**

That depends on what you mean by the word 'exercises' and why a person takes exercise at all.

**Why does a person take exercise?**

Well, people expect a lot of things from doing exercise, e.g.

(1) They believe exercise makes them physically fit
(2) They believe they would live longer, and finally
(3) They believe exercise improves their image and makes them look better.

**Is all this a false claim?**

No, I wouldn't quite say that. However, I have a quarrel with physical exercises which neglect the mind and build mainly the body.

**What are the different types of exercises?**

Technically speaking, there are three types:

1. Dynamic or isotonic
2. Isometric
3. Yogic postures

**What happens in isotonic exercises?**

In isotonic exercises the muscles shorten, but the tension in the muscles remains the same.

**Can you name some of these exercises?**

Yes, walking, cycling, swimming, running, jogging, bench stepping, skipping, etc.

## What happens in isometric exercises?

In isometric exercises, the length of the muscle does not change, but the tension increases.

## Any example?

Yes, of course. The best example is weight lifting. Similarly, when you push your hands against a wall, you can feel the tension in the muscles of your arm.

## What are the effects of different types of exercises?

Isotonic exercises increase the work of the cardiovascular system, but if performed regualrly in optimum quantity they improve physical fitness. Isometric exercises build up the muscle mass and are mainly useful for building of the muscles of the body but they do not improve stamina and physical endurance. The danger is that they can impose a severe strain on the cardiovascular system. Isometric contraction of even small muscles of the hands can increase B.P. to very high levels, and therefore, isometric exercises are considered undesirable, particularly for patients of cardiovascular diseases and are not recommended for physical training.

Yogic postures and breathing exercises unlike physical exercises (isotonic as well as isometric) do not strain the cardiovascular system and improve physical fitness and endurance. Therefore, they are useful in both health and disease. Yogic exercises are useful for the body as well as the mind. They change the reaction of the body to the day to day tensions which are so rampant today.

## And so the isometric exercises are no good for heart patients, is that right?

That's correct.

## You counted Yogic exercises (Postures) as one of the types of exercises, didn't you?

Yes, but there is a fundamental difference.

## What is the difference? I suppose exercises are exercises, and no matter what type?

Your question is based on a common misconception that Yogic exercises are physical exercises. Do you know that physical exercises are repetitive movements, whereas Yogic exercises involve very little movement and are only postures which are to be maintained for a period of time?

This is why they are called Yogic postures (asanas).

## Any examples?

Yes, for example Bhujangasana, Shirashasana, Mayurasana, etc. You will understand these words later on.

## So, is this why they are called postures?

Yes, quite so. Further, there are some basic differences between Yogic postures or asanas, and physical exercises.
(1) While Yogic postures tone up both the body and the mind, physical exercises affect mainly the body.
(2) In yogic postures you spend much less energy than you would in physical exercises.

## How can you say that Yogic postures tone up the mind?

Because these postures and breathing exercises help you to change the reaction to stress and thereby minimise the ill-effects of stress. These postures involve concentraion on certain parts of the body, and, therefore, the result is a toning up of both the mind and the body.

## How do you say that much less energy is spent on Yogic postures than in physical exercises?

Don't you agree that when you do physical exercises, you get exhausted? This is only because you spend a lot of energy. Comparatively, Yogic postures, when maintained for a definite period help to conserve energy and give a feeling of relaxation and exhilaration.

## How much energy is spent in Yogic asanas?

The caloric requirement in Yogic asanas varies from 0.8 to 3 calories per minute, while the caloric requirement of a physical exercise varies from 3 to 20 calories per minute.

## How is that an improvement on physical exercises?

Very naturally. Whereas heart patients are prohibited from doing physical exercises, they are permitted to practise many yogic postures. Isn't that a great advantage?

## I suppose so, but what are the main advantages?

Ah! If you know the difference between fatigue and freshness, you have the main advantage. In the first place, yogic exercises bring about a feeling of freshness and relaxation and remove physical lethargy. In the second place, yogic exercises are useful for the weak and the old people.

## But is it not true that physical exercises tone up muscles, improve the circulation of blood in the voluntary muscles, thereby giving us visibly developed muscles?

True, but yogic exercises are not meant to increase the muscle mass. In fact, yogic exercises are meant to improve the functioning of the organs.

## Can you cite any example?

Why not? Take, for example, 'Shirshasana' or 'Sarvangasana'. They both help to improve the circulation of the blood in the brain. In 'Uddiyana' we improve blood circulation in the abdominal organs and in 'Pranayama', that of the heart and the lungs.

## But physical exercises keep our bones and joints in trim condition, don't they?

Yes, they do, but Yogic exercises are so designed that they help to keep the spine flexible and the joints supple.

**Well, is there any other difference between the Yogic postures and physical exercises?**

As you know by now, Yogic exercises aim at both prevention and treatment of various diseases.

**Prevention, too? Any examples?**

There are breathing exercises, like Pranayama, including Kapalbhati, which are very effective for keeping the lungs healthy and prevent lung infections. With deep breathing air circulates to every part of the lungs, whereas with most other physical exercises, there is mainly an increase in respiratory rate.

**Would you say Yogic practices can advantageously replace physical exercises?**

Of course, they can, because Yogic practices are more beneficial as explained above. What is more, while physical exercises need a special place or equipment, Yogic practices need no such place or equipment. Indeed, Yoga is a comprehensive system to keep the body fit and the mind alert.

**Are there any principles to be observed for Yogic postures?**

Yes, of course. The very word 'posture' signifies the static nature of the exercise.

(1) The first principle of Yogic postures is that they should be practised in a slow and steady manner, and all jerks should be carefully avoided.

(2) The second principle is that having attained a final position in a particular posture, one should maintain the posture in a comfortable and relaxed manner.

(3) While maintaining the posture one should concentrate on the relaxed muscles and try to relax them further. Mind should not be allowed to wander.

(4) The fourth principle is that in attaining or maintaining the final position in any of the postures, due regard should be given to limitations set by one's age, sex and bodily condition.

**Do all these various postures have a common purpose?**

Yes, they do. The common purpose of all the postures is to establish a proper tone in the neuro-muscular system as a whole.

Another principle governing the practice of posture is the attitude accompanying the practice. To reap the maximum benefit from the postures, the practice should be regular, uninterrupted, and performed with full conviction.

**Can one start exercises irrespective of age or health?**

One should not start physical exercises without a thorough physical examination and making certain that the exercises to be undertaken would not do any harm. However, Yogic postures are generally mild and one is less likely to get into complications, but physical exercises, especially the type known as jogging, which is most popular in the Western world today, should never be undertaken unless the individual is fully evaluated by his physician. The physician should look for signs and symptons and take an electrocardiogram at rest and after exercise to detect an overt or subclinical heart disease. Even in a well-organised programme of jogging many complications have occured. The usual ones are: arthritis, spondolysis, rupture of muscles, lung infections, hernia, piles, etc. Even deaths have been reported while jogging. Therefore, one should be extra careful before embarking on a jogging programme. Moreover, if vigorous physical exercise is discontinued, one is apt to get into trouble as seen in athletes, wrestlers, etc.

**What about Yoga and longevity?**

In India which has a great heritage of Yoga, Yogic exercises are acceptable to most. These are useful for all, including the elderly, and even patients of heart disease. As regards longevity, though it is claimed that Yoga prolongs life and many yogis have a long life, scientific data on this subject are not available.

# PRINCIPLES OF YOGIC POSTURES

## Why is it that in Yogic exercises there is not much of movement as in gymnastics?

I wouldn't say there are no movements in Yogic practices, but as the very word 'posture' suggests, the Yogic practices (postures) are of a static nature.

In these postures, great emphasis is laid on 'static' stretching.

## Are these static methods as effective as the dynamic ones?

Yes, of course, they are. What is more, static stretching is safer than dynamic. It is easy to understand this, because in Yoga there is no sudden strain on the related tissues.

## Any other advantage?

Oh Yes! Many a time dynamic stretching causes severe muscle soreness, but static stretching does no such thing; on the contrary it relieves soreness where it exists.

## Would you call this the main feature of Yogic postures?

Indeed, the very *first principle* is that Yogic postures should be practised in a slow and steady manner and *all jerks* must be carefully avoided. That is not enough. The *second principle* is that, having attained the final position of a particular posture, you should *maintain the position* in as comfortable and relaxed a manner as possible.

## What actually happens when we do this?

In adopting and maintaining a posture there is a coordination between the nervous system and the muscular system involving various groups of muscles that are controlled by what we call the *tonic reflex system*.

## And what's this tonic reflex?

As the word suggests, the reflex sets up a kind of a tone in the body and influences the physical and mental behaviour.

**Are there any limitations regarding age, sex, or bodily condition?**

Indeed, there are. They constitute the third principle, viz. in attaining or maintaining the final position in any of the postures, due regard must be given to one's limitations as regards age, sex, and bodily condition.

**How does one take care of that?**

A feeling of 'pleasant pain' is a proper indication of the limit before one starts feeling discomfort. What is important is the *pattern* of the posture. All postures, although they differ from one another, serve a common purpose which is to establish a proper tone in the neuro-muscular system as a whole. In any case, it's a matter of attitude.

**How does one develop that?**

Well, it is done by keeping the practice regular, uninterrupted and performed with full conviction. When a protracted routine is undertaken it takes more time. In fact, the time involved should be well within the reach of a busy person.

**How long should this routine be?**

About 15 to 20 minutes every day would do much more good than a protracted routine undergone irregularly and interruptedly.

**But, after all, any posture is a physical one, isn't it? What part does the mind play?**

That's a very good question. During the practice of postures, mental activity is very important. The mind has to be engaged in following certain sensations produced by the posture.

**What if one doesn't feel the sensations?**

In that case, the alternative is to concentrate on following the course in breathing. That is why one closes his or her eyes during the exercise because that facilitates intensifying the feeling of the postures.

## Is the breathing activity a part of these postures?

Yes, one is immensely benefited by regulating one's breathing during postures. The guidelines to be followed are:

(1) Flexion should be accompanied by exhalation (breathing out);
(2) Extension should be accompanied by inhalation (breathing in).
(3) One must hold the breath while maintaining difficult positions.

When one has a near-normal breathing, it means that he or she performs the postures with ease, comfort, and in a relaxed manner.

## Any more points?

Yes, only one. The session of practising Yogic postures should start with a meditative pose to be maintained for a few minutes in order to compose oneself and to create an atmosphere favourable for deriving the maximum benefit from the routine.

## What about the selection of postures?

That should be based on the principle of proceeding from the simple to the difficult. The more intensive and difficult will follow later on.

# YOGA AND THE DIET

**Has our diet anything to do with Yoga?**

Yes, indeed. Modifying our diet and improving our eating habits are most essential in Yoga. As you know, Yoga is both a philosophy and a science. It is said that purity of mind depends upon the purity of the diet. A Yogi has to keep himself young and healthy.

**How does he do that? How does his diet differ from our modern simple layman's diet?**

The ancient yogi's diet consisted of pure cow's milk and fruits or roots that grow under the earth. It did not contain salt, chillies, condiments, and pungent or sour things. A good Yogi does the same thing even today.

**How about tea, coffee or alcohol?**

The yogi considers them as artificial and temporary stimulants and so he does not drink any of these. In modern life, diet may be modified according to many factors, e.g. (1) the climate, (2) the way of life, and (3) the availability of food . After all, what is needed is a set of dietary principles. Food is, of course, essential to build up our body because improper food naturally brings in illnesses of all sorts.

**Talking of our heart troubles, are you suggesting that even our heart ailments have something to do with our food habits?**

Certainly! Food plays an important part not only in the causation of coronary heart disease and high blood pressure, but also in diseases like diabetes, arthritis, constipation and what not.

**But you also talked of wrong eating habits, didn't you?**

Certainly! Besides the wrong type of food there are faults

in the eating itself — such as eating (1) too fast, (2) too much, (3) very hot or very cold, and (4) having heated discussions during meals. It isn't what you eat, but how you assimilate the food that matters.

## Then what do you really suggest?

There are some of the 'don'ts' and 'dos' — (1) Don't eat in haste, (2) you should be relaxed while eating, and (3) heated arguments can wait till you have finished eating.

## But why all that fuss?

Fuss, did you say? My friend, remember whatever you eat has to be digested and absorbed and then has to be used as energy and blood.

So it's common sense that (1) You masticate your food, you chew it before you swallow so that it can go to your stomach in easily digestable form. After all, what are the teeth for? You don't want the stomach to do what the teeth ought to do — do you? (2) Eating slowly, automatically means not eating too much. Overeating means overloading and bloating the stomach. Moreover, if you eat too much it leads to obesity and you become a fatso dragging your weight about with you and you invite all kinds of diseases — don't you?

## How does one find out when one has had enough?

You don't have to feel 'full' every time you eat — you must feel 'satisfied' rather than 'full', Yoga clearly says, eat when you feel hungry and not necessarily when it's time to eat. Again, Yoga helps you to control your intake of food.

## But, what are the advantages of doing that?

Well, there are obvious advantages such as improvement in (1) digestion, and (2) absorption. Also, the body gets better nourishment.

## People say that you must be a vegetarian if you want to start or practise Yoga. Is that true?

The ancient yogis were, of course, vegetarians, but you don't necessarily have to give up meat just because you are practising yoga. Proper food depends upon — (1) where you live, (2) what kind of life you lead, and (3) what work you do. For example, clerks and white collar people who lead sedentary life need simple and easily digestible foods.

**Is it not true that for proper nourishment, one must eat meat and eggs?**

Not at all! That's an erroneous belief. Actually meat contains few or hardly any vitamins or minerals, and is more difficult to digest. Besides fat and a lot of cholesterol, meat also contains more protein which produces what is medically known as *purine bodies* and uric acid.

**But what is the harm?        Harm? It leads to rheumatism.**

**What is the alternative then?**

A natural diet is the answer — viz. fruits, greens, milk, citrus fruit, and whole grains. These provide all the essential food elements. In fact, the aim of a yoga diet is to keep as closely as possible to natural foods.

**What exactly should be the different contents of food.**

We usually talk of *caloric content* of food.

**What does the word calorie mean?**

Calorie is actually a measure — a unit measuring heat. In terms of food it measures the energy the food supplies to the body; for example, one ounce or about 28 grammes of sugar is supposed to provide about one hundred calories.

Our food contents should consist of — 10 to 15% calories of fats, 10 to 15% of proteins and 75 to 80% calories of carbohydrates specially complex carbohydrates. Also bear in mind

(1)    Only 200 mg of cholestoral a day is just enough (in the west the intake is about 800 mg).

(2)  Refined carbohydrates like sugar and other processed foods (usually tinned) should be avoided.

(3)  Complex carbohydrates are good for the body. They are available in plenty in grains, vegetables, fruits. In fact they are the best.

## Why do you call them the best foods?

Because they really are the best. They give everything the body needs. Here's what they do:-

(1) They provide ample calories.
(2) They supply the necessary vitamins.
(3) They give us the minerals.
(4) They provide the dietary fibre.
(5) They give the necessary energy.

## What if one is already used to non-vegetarian food?

Well, you don't give it up suddenly. But, I suppose when a man who practises yoga, becomes spiritualy minded, his desire for flesh foods automatically diminishes. He chooses what his mind influences him to.

## One last question. How does one know whether his life style is wrong or right or rather what one's life style has done to his body, particularly to his heart and the blood vessels?

That's a professional question.

But the answer is important and so here it is.

'If you want to find out what your life-style has done to your body, particularly to the blood vessels and the heart, you can do that very easily. Get your weight, cholesterol, triglycerides, total lipids, blood pressure, ECG at rest and on exercise taken and you can find out for yourself whether your life-style has so far been right or wrong. Remember, it is possible to modify the risk factors for heart disease and thus delay or prevent the hardening of arteries and the onset of heart disease'.

# YOGA AND OBESITY

**Fat people all round us are worried about the weight they carry with them—can Yoga do anything for them?**

Yoga is meant to help to develop a perfect figure. Yoga offers a peaceful and healthy existence and it is but natural that Yoga should be of use to these unfortunate fat people. There are several reasons, good reasons, to get rid of this fat.

(1) Fatness or obesity means strain on the heart, the internal organs, the legs (meaning the ankle, the knee, the hip), in fact, the whole body. Is it any wonder then, that heart disease and other diseases like diabetes, blood pressure and arthritis are so very common ailments among the obese? In fact, deaths too are more in these fat people.

**Is it that bad?**

It certainly is. For a 10 per cent increase in weight, there is a 20 per cent increase in the chances of death, for 20 per cent increase it is 40 per cent, and for a 25 per cent increase it is as high as 75 per cent. Actually it is a *'bloody' battle of the bulge*.

**Can Yoga do nothing for them?**

I don't say so. But Yoga has no magic formula. Along with the Yogic asanas there has to be some change in the dietary habits. The important point to remember here is the fact that if you accept yoga as a whole it should alter your way of thinking and attitude towards food also.

**How does one do that?**

You don't begin with a crash programme right from the first day, and alter the food habits straightaway. There should be no strain or frustration from the change in the food habit. But, at the same time, there has to be no eating just to kill your boredom, or for the mere pleasure of eating.

A mental attitude has to be developed so that you don't cling to food as a crutch, and gradually yoga helps you to reduce your desire to eat more. In medical language, Yoga creates a state of *homeostasis*, i.e. a state when the functioning of the endocrine glands is so regulated that you lose the abnormal desire for food which the body does not need.

## Any Yogic exercises?

All yogic exercises are useful, but the following are particularly useful for weight reducing.

1. Ek Padasana,
2. Uttanapadasana,
3. Halasana,
4. Bhujangasana,
5. Ardha-Shalabhasana,
6. Vakrasana,
7. Pashchimatanasana,
8. Chakrasana,
9. Viparitakarani,
10. Sarvangasana,
11. Matsyasana,
12. Dhanurasana,
13. Yoga mudra,
14. Pavanamuktasana,
15. Parvatasana,
16. Makarasana,
17. Shavasana,
18. Uddiyanabandha,
19. Kanthasana,
20. Kapalabhati, and
21. Ujjayi.

# YOGA AND RELAXATION

## Why do people need relaxation?

What a question? Don't you think eight to ten hours of work a day must be followed by a period of relaxation?

If not, why has nature ordained that there shall be 'sleep' after a waking period?

## If, then, sleep is prescribed by nature, why do you need the yogic form of relaxation, whatever that may mean?

Now you are talking. Ask yourself if 'sound sleep' is ever possible with the fast pace of life, particularly in big cities. In fact, this pace is destructive. People keep running about in a frenzy and hardly find time to sit down and think or read a book or even listen to music.

## But where is the time for all this, when one has to work hard to make a living?

Well, that is the trouble. It is wrong to think that we cannot spare time. It is not so much the lack of time as the feeling that there is no need for such relaxation, which is the cause of this mad rush. This results in most people visiting their psychiatrists for treatment of their mental tension.

## Anyway, the modern man does make money with this sort of 'rush' life, doesn't he? Will it not help him during his period of retirement?

Money made in a life of such tension will leave him no life of retirement. A life of 'rush rush' is a life of tension, nervousness, and anxiety. Sleepless nights follow and the next day's life is one of depression.

## True, but modern science has also given us tranquillizers and sleeping pills, and these help us to relax, don't they?

Man lives in a fool's paradise if he lives in the world of sleeping pills and tranquillizers which bring an apparent respite but no cure. He only becomes dependent on them. The problem has to be tackled at the root. *Man must learn to relax.*

**Where modern science has failed, are you suggesting that Yoga will succeed?**

My friend, real yogis realised hundreds of year ago that the human mind functions best in a state of relaxation. Therefore, apart from physical exercises, Yoga has prescribed various techniques for relaxation.

**Does relaxation not mean deliberately idling away one's time in a kind of mental inertia?**

I see, you ventilate the viewpoint of many who wrongly identify relaxation with idleness or laziness, or even mental inertia as you put it.

Actually, relaxation is a breathing space in the rush of daily living. This breathing space is necessary to prepare the body for greater energy and clearer vision. It is strange, but even a change of work brings about relaxation, just as a change of crop in a field brings about greater fertility or better use of land.

**Is that why people do not feel exhausted after a vigorous game of tennis or badminton at the end of a hard day's work?**

Yes, that is one form of relaxation, but the yogic way is quite different, quite distinct, and really rewarding.

**What is this yogic way?**

The first step is relaxing the body—I mean, consciously for a few minutes. After sufficient practice you will discover that this earned relaxation becomes a part of life throughout the day. People who relax in this manner have a wonderful experience.

**What makes it wonderful?**

It is wonderful because:

(1) Not only does the body feel relaxed but also the mind, which is freed from material things outside its earthly

shell, as it were.

(2) Secondly, it makes you aware of the rich inner life you begin to experience.

(3) **Thirdly, it makes you realise the importance of deliberately slowing down when it is so necessary.**

## When and where is it possible to relax?

Well, perhaps you already know that a quiet room, not much lighted, and of a comfortable temperature, along with the wearing of comfortable clothes is conducive to a feeling of relaxation.

## But why all this fuss?

It is not fuss, but a way to prepare the mind for inactivity. The important thing is:

(1) To forget the day-to-day worries at that time, and
(2) To keep the body absolutely motionless.

## How does that help?

It helps because when you relax you feel the body being actually attracted by the earth. In fact, the force of gravity seems (mind you, I use the word 'seems') to act on every part of the body, and each part feels heavier and heavier.

## It must be an eerie feeling, isn't it?

No, not eerie, but perhaps tingling—as you feel, when you are submerged upto your neck in a bath tub, and you suddenly drain the water out. Remember that in yogic relaxation you feel the relaxation beginning from the feet and extending towards the head.

## Why is this so?

Because the largest muscles are the easiest to relax.

**Which is the most convenient posture for relaxing the body?**

The ideal yogic posture for relaxation is the *shavasana,* about which you will learn later.

For relaxation it is not necessary to lie on your back. If you find it more convenient, you may lie on the left or the right side. There is yet another posture called the Makarasana, i.e. lying on your stomach — provided, of course, you haven't had a heavy meal. Whatever the posture, it is only when the body is 'forgotten' that you feel a sense of unbelievable relaxation.

**Frankly, what I would like to know is that, apart from this feeling of relaxation, what is the advantage to the body?**

There are tremendous advantages:

(1)   Our nerve cells get invigorated because during relaxation they are relieved of their routine burden of working. Actually, a few minutes of this form of relaxation is even so much better than long hours of so-called sleep which is mostly restless.

(2)   Above all, the state of complete body relaxation leads to the discovery of a marvellous inner world, but this, of course, can be achieved only after considerable practice.

**How long should I practice this so as to achieve this inner world of yours?**

Why do you say 'yours'? You should rather say 'ours', and you *will* achieve it if you'll only start practising. Frankly, the proper relaxation technique takes about 20 to 30 minutes to start with, and it may not be possible for you to spare so much time, but soon you'll find you can achieve the same feeling more quickly.

**How about relaxing in a sitting posture?**

After practice you will learn to relax even while sitting on a chair for a few minutes but apparently this posture for relaxation is not the ideal one, although it may be helpful.

# YOGA AS A REMEDY FOR ADDICTIONS

Why is it that man today is not so healthy nor so happy as in the days gone by? With the advance in science, particularly in the field of medicine, one would have thought he should really be much healthier and happier?

Your question is a very valid one. True, with the control of diseases through medical advances man's life expectancy has increased. The conditions of living, however, have become chaotic for various reasons, and so, instead of looking brighter, people seem to look morose and tired. This is mainly because in the stress and strain of modern life man has forgotten the basic principles of good health.

Why should he do that? There are modern amenities to solve his problems, aren't there?

True, there are modern amenities, but these do not help his mental problems. People lead fast lives. They want to make more and more money and in this process, they lose themselves. They need pills to go to sleep, they need pills to move their bowels, they need tranquillisers to keep themselves calm. Even the young take to drugs.

But these pills and drugs are effective, aren't they?

Of course, they are, but don't forget they offer only a temporary solution.

As for young people, they mislead themselves. All that they do is to seek escapism with alcohol or drugs or tobacco, but this only makes them helpless in the long run. By using them, a vicious cycle is set up and eventually they become slaves to these.

Then how can man give up all this and look after his own health?

It is here that Yoga is a great boon to civilized man. Yoga is a way of life which makes him rediscover his zest for living.

How?

By following the yogic curriculum of physical and mental exercises. For example, the physical exercises of Hatha Yoga counteract the negative psychosomatic and mental conditions which appear in the form of psychological disorders.

**Do you suggest that Yoga has medicinal values?**

That is perhaps not quite the right way of putting it. It will be more correct to say that mental conditions like anxiety, restlessness, and neurosis can be treated by yogic postures.

**What is the justification for saying that?**

Well, yogic postures influence the endocrine glands like the adrenal, the thyroid, the pancreas, etc.

All that yoga does is to stimulate these glands so as to bring about mental homeostasis.

**That's a rather difficult word.**

What I mean is that as man goes on practising Yoga, he feels more relaxed, starts thinking differently, and takes life more philosophically. And with the change in attitude he is better prepared to face the modern day stresses and strains and does not need drugs, alcohol, or tobacco as a prop.

**But you cannot deny that alcohol soothes one's nerves, can you?**

Man has used alcohol since the dawn of civilisation. In fact, every civilisation has used it only to obtain a condition of mind, known as 'euphoria' which accompanies intoxication.

Alcohol has also been used in the treatment of the sick. The great Indian Physician of the 2nd century, Charaka, has actually prescribed more than *thirteen* alcoholic brews. A world famous physician of Baghdad, Ibn Sina or Avicenna was the first to describe the effcacious properties of alcohol, very, very, long ago, indeed.

**Then why worry so much now?**

You will appreciate that every medicine has its proper

dosage. So, even a thing which has medicinal value has to be taken in the right measure. Anything, even food or medicine, if taken in excess, is harmful to the human body. So is the case with alcohol. and as the habit grows, one gets addicted to it — and this is where the danger lies.

And then there are some who take to drinking because they are unhappy, frustrated, or dissatisfied with life. They ultimately become slaves to drinking. This again is hazardous.

**But man does become sober after his heavy drinking is over, doesn't he? And if this drinking helps him to appear a little fashionable and even drowns his sorrow or removes his frustration, why not let him do it?**

My dear friend, it is now well known that when taken in excess and/or over a long time, alcohol has an adverse effect on all the systems of the human body. For example, it depresses the nervous system.

**How does that harm him?**

Well, it impairs his mental functions and even his motor performances. It leads to changes in the heart muscle, resulting in what we doctors call *cardio-myopathy*. Then, with excessive drinking his digestive system too is affected.

**In what way?**

In every way. It leads to abdominal distension, belching, and pain in the *epigastrium*.

**What is this epigastrium?**

The epigastrium is the upper part of the abdomen. Anyway, it is the liver which is harmed the most. This organ cannot function normally as the liver cells are damaged The doctors call this ailment *cirrhosis* of the liver, so common in alcoholics.

**Where does Yoga, then come in?**

Yoga helps in many ways:

(1) It can prevent a person form becoming an aloholic.

(2) It can also help a person to give up alcohol altogether.

## How?

He has to be sufficiently motivated. Remember, alcoholism is not a point of no return. An alcoholic is to be treated with patience. Sufficient time is also needed.

## Has a person to give up alcohol the moment he starts Yoga? That would be very difficult.

No! when a person starts Yoga, he need not give up alcohol all of a sudden, but withdraw from it gradually. He has to develop self-confidence. With the practice of Yoga, as he is able to stand the stress and strain of modern life he begins to depend upon his stimulant less and less till he gives it up on his own. An important point to be remembered here is that he has to learn to live the yoga way of life. By following the principles of Yama and Niyama, his mind gets disciplined, his urge to drink gets diminished, and he begins to enjoy better physical and mental health.

## How about tobacco?

That came in as late as the 10th century.

You know, it is used in several forms, like smoking, chewing paan and snuffing by millions of people throughout the world, cigarette smoking being the most common way.

## Is tobacco really harmful?

Who does not know the hazards of smoking?

Smoking too has adverse effects on all systems of the body. The respiratory system and the respiratory tract are those most affected by smoking.

## What is the exact damage?

Damage? It is disastrous! It leads to cancer of the lungs. It is also a very important risk factor in coronary heart disease and the incidence of sudden death in smokers is also high. Yes, and there is one more hazard. Excessive smoking also leads to diseases of the peripheral vessels.

**What are these?**

These are diseases of the blood vessels of the limbs. The lower limbs are most affected and the patient gets pain in his legs on walking.

**But I believe most smokers know the adverse effects of smoking and yet they do not give it up. Why is it so?**

Ah! They lack the will power to do so and this is exactly what yoga provides.

**Yoga gives us will power. Is that what you mean?**

With the practice of yoga, the mind gets trained and disciplined and this is what diminishes the urge for tobacco and gradually frees one from this injurious habit.

**If alcohol and smoking are bad, drugs surely can't be that bad. Are they?**

Drug is not a word! It's a sentence—a sentence for life, if you are not careful.

**Isn't it true that drug-taking is also a kind of fashion in modern life—particularly in the young?**

Drugs are taken for various reasons.

(1) To alleviate pain.
(2) To reduce tension.
(3) To change the mood.
(4) To counter fatigue.
(5) To be more acceptable in society.
(6) To satisfy curiosity and
(7) To tackle sexual problems.

Unfortunately, it starts in a harmless way, perhaps by way of experimentation, but ultimately one gets habituated, and becomes an addict.

**I suppose there are many kinds of drugs, aren't there?**

Yes, the most common one is heroin. They sell it in the market under various names like smack, sunaq, junk, and dope. Then there are *barbiturates* like *mandrax* and these are all medicinal names—*nembutal,, seconal, doridan* and then there are *amphetamines* (dexidrin), ·*cocaine, marijuana, hashish,* LSD, etc.

### Are they equally harmful?

No! I wouldn't say that! Each drug has its own harmful qualities. Anyway, the harm each does depends upon:

(1) its own nature
(2) the way it is taken and
(3) the quantity taken, and
(4) the duration of its use.

### What exactly do these drugs do?

Well, generally speaking, initially they produce euphoria; but, finally they lead to depression and even suicidal tendencies.

### How can one prevent drug addiction?

To prevent this addiction it is necessary to provide attractive vocational, recreational, and educational alternatives.

### And Yoga?

Of course, yoga provides an excellent alternative. It gives mental and physical training, and this helps gradually to wean the individual away from drugs.

# YOGA AND SEX

## Is it true that yoga means avoiding sex completely?

No, not at all!

(1) Some proclaim that yoga practitioners must not indulge in sex at all.
(2) There are others who think that Yoga postures make you sexy.

## Then what is the correct view of yoga and sex?

The general principles of yoga lay emphasis on a healthy body, mind and the spirit. Physical fitness and control of mind are attained by a specific type of yoga known as Hatha Yoga. It is a very practical yoga and can be fully practised by most people.

## What is the philosophy of those who advocate no sex at all?

It is true that some yogis who practise celibacy do believe that sexual desires, whether conscious or sub-conscious are destructive and so must be controlled. They somehow or other believe that if the sexual urge is suppressed, it increases the power of concentration.

## How is that possible?

Well, it's a belief that when you abstain from sex, you can concentrate more, and by this sublimation you increase the power of the mind. Unfortunately, people who are attracted by the mere physical exercise part of the Hatha Yoga, indulge in this sort of philosophy. Actually, those who look at Hatha Yoga in the right perspective realise that it is a form of complete mental and physical discipline which ultimately leads to self realisation.

## How can Yoga help to suppress sexual desires?

There are many yogic techniques to do so. Hard work is one of them. Exercise is another. Meditation and prayer are a third. Study of religious books is yet another. Some think even plain and simple food would help.

## But what about yoga asanas? Do they help?

Oh yes, they do. These asanas are:

—Bhadrasana
—Ugrasana
—Gorakshasana and others.

They all help to reduce the sexual desires.

## Is there any other philosophy?

Basically all such philosophies aim at concentration of physical and sexual energies which according to them lead to a kind of transmutation of these energies into the energies of the mind. But for that we need sublimation.

## What is sublimation?

Generally speaking, sublimation means working at a sublime or high level. It involves techniques of breath control over and above concentration, and of course yogic asanas.

## Can anyone perform these asanas?

No! Not every one. It is advisable to learn these asanas with the help of a teacher.

## Doesn't that all lead to strict observance of an ascetic disposition?

Well, whatever be the meaning of the expression to you, it is positively difficult.

**But does it mean you must neglect it and even condemn it?**

Of course not! You will do no such thing! There is no doubt that the message of yoga is not that simple, particularly for an ordinary householder.

**Message? What is the message?**

It would be a repetition of all that we have said before. It is nothing but the union of the individual spirit with the universal spirit by adopting those means which cause no harm.

**I suppose to attain this self-realisation, you must leave your home, your friends and your life itself?**

No, not at all! It does not mean taking a sanyas. It doesn't mean forgetting your responsibilities to those around you, including your family and society.

**Then what is the expected standard?**

I suppose there is such a thing as universal truth so that if one lives an unselfish or *selfless life* he has accepted the way of enlightenment. Gita has propounded various paths or 'Yogas' such as Karma Yoga, Bhaktiyoga, and Gnyan Yoga. People follow these paths in varying degrees, according to their inclinations.

**But should there be a 'No Sex' life?**

My good friend, chastity does not mean complete celibacy as such. It actually means avoiding excessive lust, unlawful lust, marital infidelity and even undue indulgence in sex.

But what is the actual philosophy of life vis-a-vis Yoga? Has any great scholar given us a clear cut way of life?

It was a great yogi Vatsyayana who in his book Kamasutra has given us a glimpse of this philosophy.

**Yes, I have heard of the word Kamasutra but what does it mean?**

Kamasutra means the act of love. The book was written hundreds of years ago.

**What does it say about man's life?**

According to Kamasutra man's life is divided into four stages.

*Stage 1:* Upto the age of 25 when strict celibacy is to be maintained and deep religious study must be undertaken.
*Stage 2:* Is from 25 to 50 years of age, when one works for material comfort and practises the act of love.
*Stage 3:* When it begins, man must revert back to religious life and finally in *Stage 4:* you begin to liberate yourself from the material bondage of desires and attachments.

**Is it difficult to observe this way of life?**

No, but it depends. The act of love including sex is not wrong at all. Sex which is healthy, free of sin and shame, is a perfectly normal, natural biological need of a healthy human being.

**Can this philosophy help to solve some of the sexual problems that worry man?**

Why not, most of the sexual problems are psychological problems. Yoga brings in tranquillity of mind. It helps to control abnormal emotional states and practices, such as excess of sexuality, masturbation, homosexuality, lesbianism, and so on.

A healthy balance between physical, emotional and sexual desires of man is what yoga cares to bring about.

## What is the Ultimate Goal?

This balance must ultimately lead to peaceful and contented living for the human race as a whole, free of all the stresses and strains which we see in the world today.

# YOGA AND BEAUTY

**Why does a woman want to look beautiful?**

A frivolous answer perhaps would be that a female wants to look beautiful so that she can attract the male. My friend, to look beautiful and attractive has been the goal of every woman since the dawn of civilisation.

**What is it that makes a person appear beautiful?**

The important attributes of a beautiful appearance are a beautiful body, a lovely complexion, and a serene face due to mental tranquillity, which yoga can give.

**Why should a beautiful body mean so much to a woman?**

Because to her a beautiful body is a symbol of her femininity. Besides pleasing the viewer's eye, it reflects the values of her life style, and spreads joy. Hasn't the poet said: "A thing of beauty is a joy for ever"? For a woman, a beautiful body is a means of rousing erotic response in her man.

**Has this the sanction of our Indian culture?**

Of course. According to the ancient Indian culture, the good qualities of a woman are beauty, character, tolerance, truthfulness, courtesy, love, and a healthy sex life. It was Keats who said, 'Beauty is truth, truth, beauty'. Anyway, for all the qualities mentioned here, it is necessary for the woman to be healthy. That is why women, particularly educated women, are attracted by yoga which helps them to develop and preserve a beautiful figure, natural grace, and mental tranquillity.

**What claims can Yoga make on the benefits a human figure derives from it?**

Yoga can help to develop poise through the acquisition of a slim, supple and graceful figure. Yoga has a beneficial effect on the glands, so that an excessive desire for food is eliminated and the body *craves* only what it needs.

## Is this not a tall claim?

Not at all. Of course, yoga does not offer a magic formula which would help you to lose the extra fat even while you keep eating, not just two but even three and perhaps four square meals a day, not to talk of snacks and a few cups of tea thrown in. However, as you practise yoga over a period of time, your excessive desire for food will diminish.

## Do you mean to say the yogic asanas do not help you to reduce your fat?

Only to a certain extent, but you need a dietetic control as well. To get the full benefit of yoga, you must make yoga a way of life.

## What does that mean?

Simple—follow the principles of yoga not as a system of physical education or culture, but as something you believe in, something which gives you an inner satisfaction.

## How can one believe in these principles?

Well, first things first. Let's understand why women put on kilos and kilos of fat.

(1) In the first place, they eat the wrong type of food.
(2) They eat more than what they need.
(3) They lose control over their appetite.
(4) They do not take any exercise.

## But why do people eat more food than they need?

They do so for various reasons:

(1) They overeat because their mental peace or tranquillity is disturbed. People need a calm mind, which yoga can give them.

(2) They go to food, as it were, for comfort.

## And the solution?

Simple again—practise yoga and just alter your eating habits, and this will bring about a gradual change. After all, it is possible to change one's attitude towards many things, and one of these things is eating. One must eat, but only to keep fit, not to keep fat!

# YOGA AND BACKACHE

**Why is it that we hear today every third man complaining of backache?**

Are you really surprised at this extremely common complaint?

**When we know the back is composed of so many bones, I thought there should be hardly any pain.**

Ah! It's not just a question of having so many bones. The structure of the back is very complex. The human spine has many joints, is full of ligaments and cartilages, all of which run a great risk when the spine is overworked or shall I say 'wrongly' worked?

**Wrongly worked? What do you mean by that?**

The majority of causes are grouped under mechanical or degenerative backache. For instance, look at the easy chairs—actually they are too easy. Next, have a look at your badly shaped car seats or even chairs on which you sit and work for hours. Remember, bad postures and fatigue together cause backache.

**Are you suggesting that these aches are just natural?**

Oh! No! These aches are caused by an unnatural position held for hours on end. Of course, there are natural backaches, too.

**Really? What are they? When are they caused?**

Well, there is the postural back pain for women during pregnancy.

**That, of course, is understandable, but such a pain is temporary, isn't it?**

Yes, the postural back pain of pregnancy usually disappears after childbirth, but mind, sometimes this pain is substituted by what we call lumbosacral pain due to childbirth itself.

### But why do old people complain of backache?

Their pain comes under the group 'degenerative changes'. These changes of the spine are almost always present after the age of 40.

### Are there no symptoms that give the warning?

Unfortunately no. These changes are not necessarily accompanied by symptoms.

### But, what causes these pains?

Scientifically speaking, they are caused by the compression of the cartilages, the soft cushioning pieces between the vertebrae.

### What about people inclined to be obese?

Yes, people suffering from obesity and even mental tension also suffer from backache. In fact, medically speaking, there are backaches due to metabolic causes.

### What is this metabolic cause?

We use this word when we talk of a process in an organism or a single cell by which nutritive material is built up into living matter or broken down into simpler substances. So, that metabolism can be constructive as well as destructive. When the metabolic products are not excreted, e.g. uric acid, it results in gout.

### Can backache be due to other causes?

Of course, there are numerous causes—psychogenic, infective, etc.

### Do you think backache can be caused by stomach ailments?

Why not? It is possible that gastro-intenstinal trouble may also be the cause.

**Is there a way to classify these backaches?**

Generally, we divide backaches into two broad divisions, acute and chronic.

**We get acute backache as a result of injury, don't we?**

Yes, indeed, but acute pain is what the housewife or gardeners and even horse riders get. Then there is the backbone fever called *dengue* which also causes acute backache.

**What about the chronic type?**

That is the backache we were talking about all the while. We call them, as you know, mechanical or degenerative and even traumatic. And don't forget, the most common cause in the modern world is bad posture and fatigue due to long sitting.

**Can't yoga come to man's aid in backaches?**

Yes, all the yogic asanas are useful but a few yogic poses and exercises are very, very useful for giving relief.

**Which are those asanas?**

It is common sense to conclude that any asana that is connected with the spine, would help. And that is a fact—the extension exercises are extremely useful. Yogic asanas like Bhujangasana, Naukasana, and Shalabhasana are most useful.

**Isn't it true that old people generally suffer from backache and arthritis?**

Yes, they do, but if yogic exercises are started early in life you can prevent arthritis and backache which are the crippling degenerative diseases of the present generation.

# POINTS TO REMEMBER BEFORE STARTING YOGIC ASANAS

**These postures or asanas that you talked about—are there any specific points to remember, when practising them ?**

Oh yes ! Quite a few. They are based on when, where, how and under what conditions, when and when not to practise them, and so on.

**Are you suggesting that yoga should be practised at a fixed time ?**

That would be clear to you if you take into consideration the following points:

### 1. *Point of time*

If in the midst of doing anything worthwhile you feel uneasy because of the urge to go to the toilet, what would you do first ?

If yoga practice has to bring about harmony between the body, the mind, and the soul, it follows that you should feel easy.

Therefore the right time to practise it is the morning time after you have cleared your bowels and emptied your bladder—don't you think so ?

**Does it mean yoga must be practised in the morning only ?**

It does not mean that yoga asanas cannot be practised in the evenings. As long as you practise them with complete ease, it does not matter whether it is morning or evening.

### 2. *Point of place:*

If you are in the midst of doing a thing in which you are interested, you would not like to be disturbed—is not that true ?

Therefore, if yoga means concentration. the need for not being disturbed, is all the greater. Hence, Yoga has to be practised in a quiet room.

### At the same place always ?

Not necessarily and perhaps not always possible, either. Yes, if you are lucky enough to find a particular place free for you, it would be advisable to stick to it because when yoga is practised at the same time and at the same place, your body and mind get conditioned to it.

### (3) *Point of clothing*

It is commonsense that man does work freely and comfortably if he is not overclothed or uncomfortably clothed.

Yoga too has to be practised in clothes that are comfortable.

### Do we have to put on our gymnastic clothes ?

No harm, but remember yoga is not an exercise. In yoga you don't strain at all, as you do when taking physical exercises. Therefore free, loose, clean, and decent clothes are just what you need. In fact, clothes depend upon the season and one can wear as the temperature permits.

### (4) *Point of Equipment*

In an activity which depends on the body and the mind and your inner self, if I may say so, you do not need any extraneous tools or equipment.

### Don't you need a quilt or mattress or something ?

Of course not ! Since you sit on the ground for the asanas, all that you need is a little mat or a folded blanket to keep you protected against the cold and the hard surface of the floor.

### (5) *Point of Food*

Can one do anything well on a heavy stomach ? Of course not. Well, yoga is no exception.

### When must we practise yoga ?

In the morning on an empty stomach or say four to five

hours after a heavy meal or at least two hours after a light meal.

## And what about bath ?

### (6) Point of Bath

It is quite refreshing to do anything creative or interesting after one's bath, so it is with yoga. But there are some who would like to have a bath after the yogic asanas. It depends.

## (7) Special points to be careful about

Yes, women should avoid asanas during the first few days of menstruation.

By the same token, asanas must be avoided during pregnancy. However, during the first few months some asanas can be practised provided they are done under the guidance of a yoga expert.

You must feel refreshed after yogic asanas and not tired or exhausted. If you do feel tired then you are mixing it up with normal exercises. If you do the asanas correctly, you will feel refreshed and not tired.

It is a good thing to help your body to get accustomed to the whole yogic process, if you do the asanas:

   (i) in the same order,
  (ii) with a few seconds of rest or relaxation between two asanas,
 (iii) **with no haste at all and without racing against time**,
  (iv) with measured counts and without quickening pace for want of time, and
   (v) with complete relaxation at the end by a special kind of asana known as 'Shavasana' about which you will learn later on.

## Any special warning ?

Yes, when you are in a posture, you bring into play certain unused muscles. In such a case there may be a feeling of stiffness, in the beginning.

Don't worry about that, for that is only a temporary phenomenon. The stiffness will go away in a few days.

# YOGIC CURRICULUM

**Who was the great exponent of yoga and what was his contribution to yoga training ?**

The great exponent of yoga, who lived in the second century B.C. was Patanjali and he described eight steps in yoga training.

**On what is his curriculum based ?**

The yogic curriculum is based on a combination or synthesis of both the physical and mental aspects. Of course, the curriculum is graded.

**Are there any restraints in the course ?**

Yes, there are some. They are known as 'Yama'. There is a code of ethics, and yoga insists on the daily practice of this code.

**Why is this practice necessary ?**

Well, it is necessary as a disciplinary training till the whole process of normal elevation becomes a part of one's life and living.

**But what are the contents of this code ?**

The contents are summed up in certain values—positive and negative.

**And, pray, what are they ?**

They are: (1) Non-violence known as 'Ahimsa' as you perhaps know, this was Mahatma Gandhi's principal value.
(2) Truthfulness or Satyam—a value of our national symbol.
(3) Non-stealing called 'Asteya'.
(4) Sex-control—Brahmacharya, a value worth cultivating in moderation.
(5) 'Aparigraha'—or control over the desire to hoard wealth—a value so badly needed these days.

## But what about the observances?

The observances or 'Niyama' as they are called, include:

(1) Purity of body and mind—they call it 'Shauch'.

(2) Contentment—we call it 'Santosh', don't we ? The next is,

(3) Self-discipline, they use the word 'Tapas'

(4) Swadhyaya—Self study, 'Swa' meaning self, and finally

(5) Resignation or surrender to God for which is the phrase 'Ishwar Pranidhana'.

## But actually of what good are the asanas to the body or to the mind and who can practise these ?

First and foremost, doing the various asanas means increasing blood circulation to the vital organs like the heart, brain, lungs, kidneys, endocrine glands. Secondly, the caloric requirement of these asanas is very low and so they could be prescribed even to those who are forbidden to practise standard physcial exercises and thirdly, these asanas are such that they can be learnt and practised at any age.

## What is Patanjali's definition of an asana ?

An asana, according to Patanjali, is that bodily posture which conforms to steadiness but is at the same time pleasant and comfortable. In other words, the pose must make you steady and also create feeling of pleasure and comfort.

In our sacred books, the Vedas, and Upanishads, it is clearly mentioned that it is impossible to get mental harmony without a steady, comfortable and balanced pose.

## Can you lump all the asanas together in the same category?

Actually asanas are of two types:

(1) Cultural and

(2) Meditative

The cultural ones are for the specific purpose of regulating the nervous and endocrine system, while the meditative poses are for the control of the mind.

The beauty about yogic asana is that when one has learnt an asana properly, he or she doesn't need a conscious effort to maintain a pose.

**But what about the breathing practises ?**

The system of physical culture accompanied by respiratory and nervous control enables an individual to regulate his biological functions by what they call bioenergy control or control of prana.

**Does it mean that pranayama enables one to control his biological functions ?**

Yes, but in such a way that it improves cardio-respiratory function, thus ultimately preparing him for true meditation.

**What about our sense-organs ? What controls them ?**

I am glad you mentioned that. Actually what follows pranayama is 'Pratyahara', i.e. the control of sense organs. And now, we come to something difficult to understand, though not impossible. The pratyahara, is actually the process of abstraction. It is the link between the outer form of yoga, i.e. 'bahiranga' and the inner one, i.e. 'antaranga'.

**It is rather difficult to understand. But tell me, how is it done, anyway?**

It is done by a training which helps one to withdraw the mind from the objects of its desire. You want a thing, but you are so trained that you resist wanting it.

**Is it really possible to train your mind that way ?**

Why not ? All that you do is relax, visualise and centralise, and with sufficient will-power you free yourself from emotional and environmental distractions. In other words, it prepares one for further and further control of the mind.

**But all that must need a terrific sense of concentration ?**

Oh yes, concentration or 'Dharana' or focussing is the main thing. Actually 'Dharana' enables the person to fix his mind and to focuss it on certain points to the exclusion of all others. After 'Dharana', the next step is 'Dhyana'. It means contemplation of the self (Atma). And all this is done when he is alone, and then comes 'Samadhi'.

**'Samadhi' ? What does that mean ?**

In common parlance we call it meditation or being 'absorbed' deeply. It's the final stage—the final stage of yoga, where the individual reaches the climax of physical, mental, and spiritual evolution. Do you know what they call this state ?

**No, what do they?**

This is a state of super consciousness. Some call it a state of immense joy and peace and concrete self realisation.

**But isn't it all mystic?**

May be, according to some; some do refer to Samadhi as a state of mysticism, but the great pandits in yoga have proved that it is not so. They aver that it is the end result of intensive training when the person attains the final bliss.

# SURYANAMASKAR

The word 'Suryanamaskar' is easy to understand, 'Surya' means the Sun, while 'Namaskar' means 'Salutation'—isn't that so ?

Yes, you are right, but remember Suryanamaskar is *not* a yogic exercise.

**Then why talk about it at all ?**

It has been included here, because it has a value in the maintenance and also promotion of health. Besides, it has a long tradition of its own as a system of exercise serving the need of a dynamic exercise with controlled breathing.

**But what is the connection between yoga and Suryanamaskar ?**

Well, there is a direct link. Yoga asanas need flexibility of the spine and the limbs. The positions in Suryanamaskar resemble some asanas and contribute to this flexibility. Therefore, they could be of help in the practice of asanas.

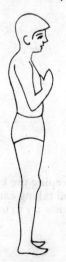

**How does one do this Suryanamaskar ?**

There are several stages:

*Stage 1:* You stand erect with folded hands.

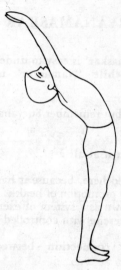

*Stage 2:* You inhale as you raise your arms above the head and bend backward.

**And then ? Stage 3 ?**

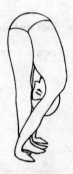

*Stage 3:* You exhale, bending forward. Keeping the knees straight, you place your hands on the ground taking care to see that they are in line with your feet. You now try to touch the knees with your forehead.

**But that must be difficult—mustn't it ?**

I said 'Try' to touch. In the beginning your knees may be slightly bent, but as you practise, you find that your head can touch them.

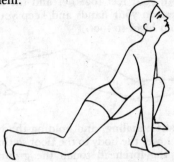

*Stage 4:* Take a big backward step, with the right leg.

## What about the hands ?

They will be kept vertical with your elbows unbent but of course, your left foot must be firmly on the ground, with the head bending backwards.

## Would it be like a sort of backward arch ?

No, not quite, but the body does assume an inclined position with the head bent backward. As for the left knee, it should be between the hands.

## What about breathing ?

I was coming to that.

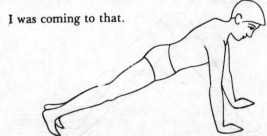

*Stage 5:* You inhale and move your left leg backward and place it alongwith the right leg.

### You mean the starting position ?

Yes, keep both your feet together and the knees off the ground. You rest on your hands and keep your body in a straight line from head to foot.

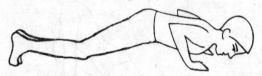

*Stage 6:* You start exhaling, and holding the breath, bend your arms, and lower the body to the floor so that the knees, the chest, and the forehead touch the ground. The abdominal region is kept raised, and if possible the nose is kept off the floor.

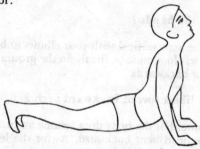

*Stage 7:* You start inhaling, and pushing your body forward through the two arms, bend backwards to extend the spine as much as possible.

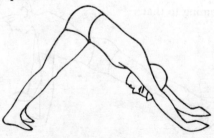

*Stage 8:* You exhale and lift your body and hips, keeping the feet and heels flat on the floor.

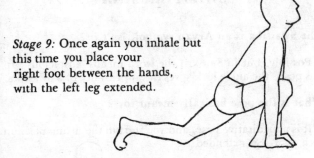

*Stage 9:* Once again you inhale but
this time you place your
right foot between the hands,
with the left leg extended.

**And where does one look ?**

You look up—slightly.

**And when do we exhale ?**

*Stage 10:* You exhale as you bring your left foot forward and
keep it with the right one between the hands assuming the
same position which you first found difficult in stage 3
above.

*Stage 11:* And now you inhale, but once again you stand
erect with folded hands exactly as you began in stage 1.
This completes one round of Suryanamaskar

**And how many rounds do we practise?**

That depends on your capacity. Usually 12 such rounds
are practised. But the number of rounds could be more or
less.

**May I know how all this is advantageous to the body ?**

Sun salutation or the Suryanamaskar helps you as
follows:

1. It contributes to muscular strength.
2. It gives you a feeling of endurance as well as exhilaration.
3. It makes your spine and your limbs flexible.
4. It improves breathing capacity.
5. It reduces your, abdominal fat.

# SWASTIKASANA

**The Swastika is an Aryan symbol, isn't it ?**

Possibly, but in Sanskrit the word means 'auspicious'. In this pose, 'the ankle lock' gives the appearance of a Swastika.

**What is the pose basically meant for ?**

It is a meditative pose, and you start in the sitting position with your legs extended.

**What are the stages ?**

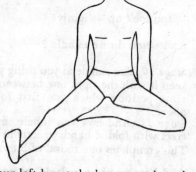

*Stage 1* : Bending your left leg at the knee you place the left foot against the right groin, the sole of that foot being in close contact with the right thigh.

*Stage 2* :

Place your right foot between the left thigh and the left calf, the two feet being now between the calf and the thigh muscles.

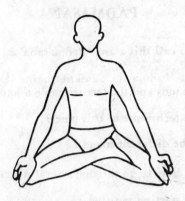

*Stage 3-4* : With your hands placed comfortably on the two knees you sit erect with your eyes closed.

*Stage 5* : You may maintain this pose for as long as you feel comfortable.

This asana may be done starting with the right leg, instead of the left.

### Any 'Dos'?

Adjust the toes between the thighs and the calves comfortably.

### Any 'Don'ts'?

Positively ! no hunch back and no bending at the loins !

# PADMASANA

**Why do you call this asana 'Padmasana' ?**

The word 'Padma' in Sanskrit means 'Lotus'. In this asana, the hands and the feet resemble a lotus flower.

**What is the technique of this pose ?**

**What are the different stages ?**

Well, you have to go through several stages.

**What is the starting position ?**

You sit with your legs fully extended forward but kept together.

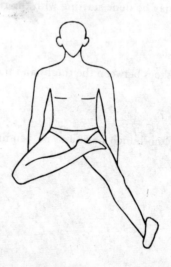

*Stage 1 :*   (a) Bend your right leg at the knee joint.
           (b) Place it on the left thigh, as near the abdomen as possible, but see that the sole is up-turned.

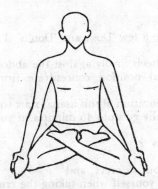

*Stage 2* : Do the same with your left leg, placing it on the right thigh.

*Stage 3* : Adjust your heels in such a way that they meet almost in the middle, just above the pubic bones.

## What about the hands ?

With your spine erect, see that the palms are on your knees.

## Anything else ?

Yes. *Stage 4:* Close your eyes and concentrate on breathing in and out.

## How does one unwind oneself from this position ?

The same slow way you wind yourself in.

*Stage 5* : (a) Withdraw your left foot from the right thigh, stretching it forward.

(b) Next, the right foot, again stretching it forward.

## That means, coming back to the starting position ?

Yes indeed.

### Any cautions ?

Yes, there are a few 'Dos', and 'Don'ts'. First the 'Dos'.

1.  Press your heels firmly against the abdomen.
2.  In the final position concentrate firmly with every breath.
3.  As for the duration of this asana, start with five minutes and gradually go upto 45 minutes, if you can.

### And the 'Don'ts' ?

1.  Don't sag, but sit erect, and
2.  Don't force yourself when taking the cross-legged position.

### Any variations in this position ?

Yes, there is an advanced variation: viz.
Padmasana, made up of a combination of two bandhas:
1.  The Jalandhara Bandha and
2.  The Mula Bandha.

### What are the advantages of this asana ?

1.  As this asana deals with the pelvic region, the first advantage is free and increased circulation of the blood in this region.
2.  You experience a feeling of inner peace.
3.  Since you sit erect, the defects, if any, of the spine are corrected.
4.  Since you concentrate firmly in this asana, it is a good asana for meditation.

### Won't these postures cause pain in the knees ?

No, not unless you are suffering from arthritis, in which case you must consult your doctor *before* practising the asana.

N.B.    If you have to learn some other Yogic Asanas for which Padmasana is the starting position, it will be desirable for you to learn this asana beforehand.

# EKA PADASANA

**I suppose the word 'Pada' suggests that this asana has something to do with the leg—hasn't it ?**

Yes, Eka Padasana is a synonym for alternate leg raise.

**How does one start ?**

As usual, you lie supine with your feet together and hands placed on the sides.

**And the technique ?**

It is in the following stages:

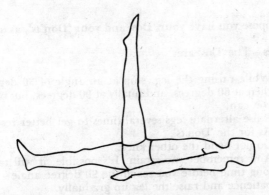

*Stage 1 :* Inhale and raise one leg slowly upto an angle of 90 degrees without bending if possible,

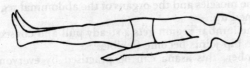

*Stage 2 :* Exhale, and lower the leg.

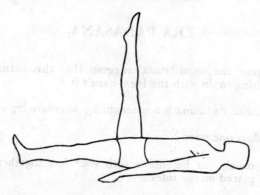

*Stage 3 :* Do the same with the other leg.

*Stage 4 :* You are back to the starting position.

**I suppose you have your 'Dos' and your 'Don'ts', as usual.**

Yes—The 'Dos' are:

1. While raising the leg, stop at an angle of 30 degrees, then at 60 degrees, and finally at 90 degrees, but only if you can.
2. Raise alternate legs several times to get better results.
As for the 'Don'ts':
1. Do not bend the other knee.
2. And remember, no strain. It's possible, it will take a long time before you reach the 90 degree angle—have patience and raise the leg up gradually.

**What are the advantages ?**

The beneficial effects of this asana are:

1. The muscles and the organs of the abdominal region are toned up.
2. The lumbar region gets a steady pull and consequently the hip joints become flexible.
Remember, this asana can be practised by everyone with benefit.

# UTTANAPADASANA

**Since the word 'Pada' is there, I presume this asana has something to do with our feet ?**

Clever, indeed. Actually it has to be done with both legs raised. It is called 'supine leg raise'.

**But we did talk earlier of 'Eka Padasana'—didn't we ?**

Yes, and this is similar to the Eka Padasana except that in this asana both the legs are raised simultaneously. Now I am sure it is clear to you that the Sanskrit word 'Uttana' means 'raise' and 'Pada' means 'legs'.

**How do we start ?**

*Stage 1 :* Lie supine with your hands on the sides and the feet together.

*Stage 2 :* Inhale and hold the breath. Then slowly raise both the legs without bending the knees and stop at a 30 degree angle.

*Stage 3 :* Extend the angle to 60 degrees, and then further to 90 degrees.

**Once again pause ?**

Yes, of course, just for a few seconds, and then exhale and lower the legs first to a 60-degree angle and then to a 30-degree one.

**And then again further down ?**

Yes, till both the legs are brought to the ground and you then relax.

**Anything important to remember ?**

Of course.

1. Raising as well as lowering of the legs must be slow, and according to your capacity.
2. Repetition of this exercise will give you good results.
3. If you are suffering from *'lordosis'*

**What's that ?**

That's an anterior curvature of the spine in the lumbar region. If you are suffering from that, you put some padding under the lumbar region to remove or lessen the strain or in the alternative, you raise your legs from the bent knee position, to start with.
4. Don't bend the knees, and as for the buttocks, they must *not* be raised.

**I suppose the benefits are the same as with Eka Padasana ?**

How very true ! Yes, they are, and on a greater scale, but basically they tone up and strengthen the *psoas* and the abdominal muscles.

# NAUKASANA

**Has this something to do with boating ?**

In a way this asana resembles the form of a boat, and hence the word Naukasana.

**Does one have to be supine ?**

Yes, that's the way to start, but then follow these stages:

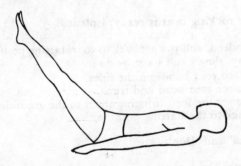

*Stage 1:* Inhale and raise the legs together till they are at about a 45-degree angle, taking care not to bend them.

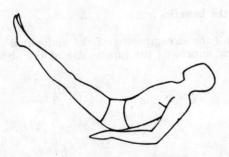

*Stage 2:* Also, raise your head and even the trunk to the same angle, viz. 45 degree.

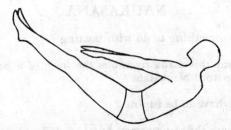

*Stage 3:* Stretching the hands forward, maintain this position.

## And the rocking boat is ready, isn't it ?

Yes, indeed, and you get back to your starting position the usual way, slowly and stage by stage.
1. Place your hands on the sides.
2. Lower your head and trunk.
3. Lower the feet, bringing them to the ground, and so, back to the starting position.

## The 'Dos' and 'Don'ts'?

The only 'Do' is to try and get the maximum contraction of the abdominal muscles by comfortably adjusting the angle of the raised legs and trunk.

And the only 'Don't' is: Don't bend your knees.

## What are the benefits ?

Again, it's the strengthening of the abdominal muscles and thereby improving the functioning of the abdominal organs.

# VIPARITAKARANI

## What is 'Viparita' ?

It means topsy turvy. Actually Viparita Karani means *'Inclined topsy turvy pose'*.

As the word topsy turvy suggests, in this pose, the position of the body is inverted, the head being on the ground and the legs up.

## I suppose we start by lying supine ?

Yes, of course, but there are definite stages.

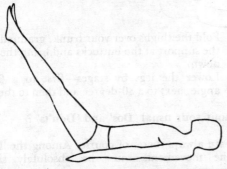

*Stage 1 :* Raise both your legs and hold them at a 30-degree angle without bending at the knees.

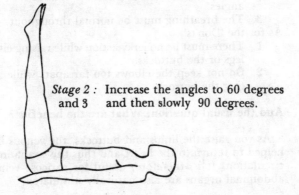

*Stage 2 :* Increase the angles to 60 degrees
and 3 and then slowly 90 degrees.

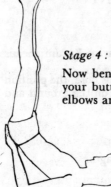

*Stage 4 :*

Now bend the legs towards your head, and raise your buttocks with both the hands, bringing the elbows and the legs in a vertical line.

*Stage 5 :* Fold the thighs over your trunk, gradually remove
*Stage 6* the support at the buttocks and bring the buttocks down.

*Stage 7 :* Lower the legs by stages—first to a 60-degree
*8   &9* angle, next to a 30-degree and then to the ground.

### What about your usual 'Dos' and 'Don'ts' ?

These are always there, of course. Among the 'Dos':
1. The movements must be absolutely slow and gradual.
2. Beginners may raise the legs straight to 90 degrees without maintaining them at the 30 and 60-degree angles.
3. The breathing must be normal throughout.

As for the 'Don'ts',
1. There must be no jerky action while raising either the legs or the buttocks.
2. Do not keep the elbows too far apart while supporting the buttocks.

### And the usual question: What are the benefits ?

As you raise the limbs and buttocks, the venous blood is helped to return to the heart and thus this asana improves circulation. It is, therefore, useful for varicose veins. The abdominal organs are also naturally stimulated.

# SARVANGASANA

**From what little I know, doesn't 'Sarva' mean 'all' ?**

Yes, 'Sarva' means 'all', 'anga' means 'body' and so 'Sarvangasana' is an asana that affects all the parts of the body.

**From the diagram here I see that this is also a topsy turvy pose, isn't it ?**

Indeed it is, though not quite. Let's get on to it.

**We start the usual way, don't we ?**

Yes, i.e., lie on your back, rest the hands on the sides of your body and the palms on the floor keeping the legs together, and stretched out. And you know what to do next. Raise both the legs from the hip joint.

**How high should they be raised ?**

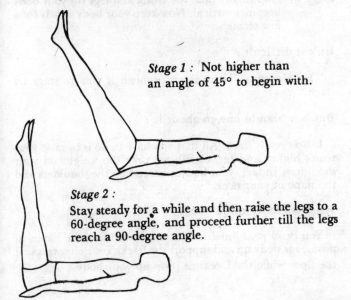

*Stage 1 :* Not higher than an angle of 45° to begin with.

*Stage 2 :*
Stay steady for a while and then raise the legs to a 60-degree angle, and proceed further till the legs reach a 90-degree angle.

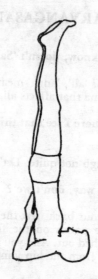

*Stage 3 :*  And finally raise the trunk and legs till your body
           becomes vertical. Now keep your body steady for a
           few seconds.

### Isn't it difficult ?

That depends. There is no problem if you go stage by
stage.

### But how should one go about it ?

It isn't really hard. All that you have to do is to raise your
trunk higher and higher till you take the weight on your
shoulders. In fact, your body must rest on the shoulders and
the nape of your neck.

### What is the technique used ?

You bend your forearms at the elbows using the hands to
push your body up and support the back. Your elbows touch
the floor while the forearms prop up your body.

**I suppose we lower the legs in order to come back to the starting position.**

Yes, you do that with or without stopping at the 45-degree or the 60-degree position. And when you do, remember:

1. to let your movement be steady and relaxed at every stage,
2. to breathe slowly but regularly,
3. to make sure that the lower part of your back lies flat against the ground. If there is a hollow, support it with a folded towel.
4. In the final position, the nape of your neck should be flat on the ground and your head should not be raised (the chest should be brought to touch the chin and not the chin to the chest).
5. During the return, bring your legs down gradually in the same way (in reverse order) as you raised them, and do not raise your head from the carpet.
6. To start with, Sarvangasana may be practised just for a few seconds. Later on, it can be maintained for two or three minutes.
7. If you cannot reach the vertical position gradually, raise your legs straightaway to 90-degree angle without pausing at 45 and 60-degree angles.

**What are the 'Don'ts' ?**

1. While raising the legs, do not do so with a jerk.
2. After the asana is completed, do not get up suddenly.

**What are the beneficial effects ?**

1. The asana is useful in cases of *varicose veins*.
2. It is also helpful in cases of swelling of the lower extremities (retention of water) from a non-cardiac cause.
3. It improves posture and carriage.
4. It is useful in cases of *insomnia*. It tones up the digestive and the liver functions. It helps to maintain a youthful look.

## Are there any contra-indications ?

1. Patients with ailments of the spine, particularly of the lumbar and cervical regions should practise this asana only after consulting a doctor.
2. Patients who have symptoms of less blood supply to the brain like fainting, giddiness, headache, etc., should consult their physician.
3. Avoid if you have:
   (a) Ear, teeth, and gum infections
   (b) Heart disease
   (c) Thyroid dysfunction
   (d) Hypertension
   (e) Sinusitis
   (f) Diseases of the eyes like detachment of retina, conjunctivitis, etc. However, it can be practised by persons with defective vision.

# SHIRSHASANA

**Shirsha is the head, of course, isn't it ?**

Yes, 'Shirshasana' is the head pose—once again a topsy turvy pose.

**How do we start this time ?**

We begin by kneeling. And now the stages, which are quite a few.

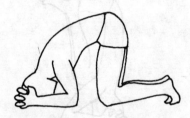

*Stages:*
1. Take a soft cushion or a four-fold blanket, interlock the fingers of your hands and place your elbows on the cushion or blanket—say about 30 cms apart.
2. Place the centre of the head on the ground taking the support of the fingerlock.

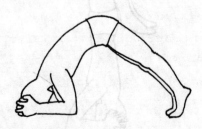

3. Raise the knees from the ground and straighten them.

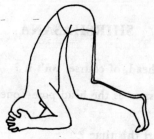

4.  Bring the feet closer to the body.

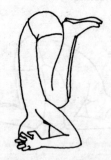

5.  With your weight on the elbows, and the abdominal
    muscles contracted, raise the feet off the ground.

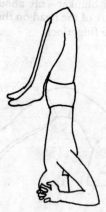

6.  Keep the knees bent, but straighten the thighs.

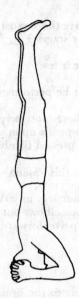

7. Straighten the knees and maintain the whole body in a vertical position.

## Now the return journey begins, doesn't it ?

Yes, it does. On your return journey the first thing to do is to —

8. Bend at the knees.
9. Lower the thighs, bringing the knees closer to your chest.
10. Touch your feet to the ground.
11. Slide your feet away from the body and straighten the knees.
12. Bring your knees to the ground.
13. Raise your hands from the ground.
14. Lift the fingerlock and loosen your fingers to return to the starting position.

**Any cautions ? I am sure there must be many, considering that there are so many stages ?**

Well, there are quite a few:

1. All actions must be performed slowly and with normal breathing.
2. At each stage there must be perfect balance.
3. Your balance depends upon your elbows and so the elbows must be pressed firmly.

As for the 'Don'ts'

1. Don't practise this asana immediately after a vigorous exercise.
2. Avoid raising your legs in jerky manner.
3. Don't spread your elbows out too much.
4. Don't push the pelvis forward.

**And the benefits ?**

These are evident.

1. Full blood supply to the brain, the nervous system, the sensory organs, the endocrine glands, and the digestive organs.
2. A good exercise that strengthens the vertebral column.
3. In this pose, gravity helps the venous blood to return to the heart — a positive help in the case of varicose veins.

*Cautions:*

Only normal and healthy persons should practise this pose. All those suffering from eye, nose, throat, and heart complaints should consult their doctors before practising this asana.

# MATSYASANA

**The word 'matsya' sounds like fish. Is it a fish pose ?**

Indeed, it is. What is more, if you practise the pose, you can float like a fish. Actually it does help one to float in water and so this asana is called matsyasana, the synonym being 'supine backward curve'.

**Are there many stages for this pose ?**

Not many, but you use some of your basic asanas. For example, you sit with legs extended and then —

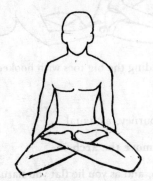

*Stage 1* :  Padmasana and

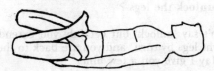

*Stage 2* :  With the help of your elbows lie on your back.

**What is the idea ?**

Well, you need your back to form an arch, don't you ? and so,

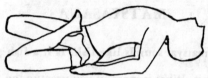

*Stage 3* : With the help of your hands turn your head
          backward.

**How do we maintain the pose ?**

That is done in

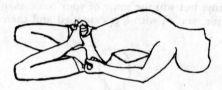

*Stage 4* : By holding the big toes with hooked index fingers.

**And then ?**

The reverse journey, as usual.

**I suppose we remove the arch ?**

Yes, you do so, and as you lie flat you naturally leave hold
of the big toes.
Then comes the time to sit up with the help of the elbows.

**And then unlock the legs ?**

I wouldn't say 'unlock' but cetainly you extend the left
and the right legs by turn, and you are back to the starting
position. May I give you a few hints.

**Please do.**

Maintain the maximum arch—keeping the elbows bent.
Don't strain while maintaining the pose. I mean, keep it
only as long as you feel comfortable.

**I have a question—If padmasana is not possible, would any other sitting position do ?**

Why not ? This asana can be practised as long as you keep your palms down under thighs.

**Why does this pose somehow remind `me of the Sarvangasana ?**

That's because it is complementary to it. And that's also why it improves the flexibility of the spine. Further it contributes to better functioning of the organs within the abdominal region. This, of course, is bound to happen because the asana gives a steady stretch to the abdomen, and since you use the whole spine, it is useful for the stiffness of the neck and cervical spine. If you have stiffness of the spine it is desirable to consult your doctor before starting this asana, so as to determine the nature of your ailment.

# HALASANA

**I see a plough here. Is that why it is called Halasana ?**

The word 'Hala' in Sanskrit means 'plough' and when the body is supine and backward stretched it takes the shape of a plough or 'hala' and hence the phrase Halasana.

**I suppose we begin as in Sarvangasana which we have done before—don't we ?**

Yes, lying flat on your back and with your palms on the floor, you follow these stages.

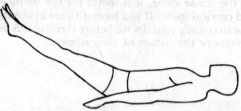

*Statge 1:* Raise both your legs in a steady movement upto a 30° angle and maintain the pose for a few seconds.

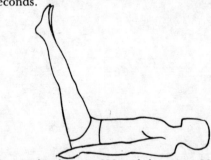

*Stage 2 :* Next, raise them to 60° and then upto 90° or the vertical position, and pause.

**Where is the plough here ?**

The plough is just half way and so we call this pose 'Ardha-Halasana', 'ardha' meaning 'half'.

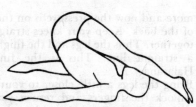

*Stage 3* : If you can, take the legs towards the head, without bending the legs, and then slowly raise the hips and the lower part of your back.

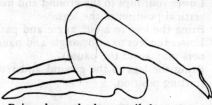

*Stage 4* : Bring down the legs until the toes touch the floor beyond your head.

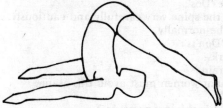

*Stage 5* : Push the legs further from your head, and maintain this stage for few seconds.

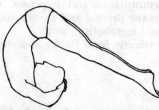

*Stage 6* : Remove the hands from the sides of your body and take them beyond the head. Make a finger-lock and, taking support of this at the head, push toes still further so that the back is bent

more and now the pressure is on the upper part of the back. Keep your knees straight and close together. Thus the legs and the thighs must be in a straight line. This is the final stage of Halasana.

*Stage 7* : Bring the legs a little closer to your head.

*Stage 8* : Unlock the fingers and return your hands to their original extended position on the sides.

*Stage 9* : Draw the legs closer to your head.

*Stage 10* : Bring the legs still closer to your head.

*Stage 11* : Lower your hips to the ground and maintain the vertical position of the legs.

*Stage 12* : Bring the legs to a 60° angle and pause.

*Stage 13* : Lower the legs to a 30° angle and pause. (Beginners may avoid the pause).

*Stage 14* : Bring the legs to the ground and return to the starting position.

## What are the 'Dos' and 'Don'ts'

First the 'Dos':
1. Bend the spine very carefully and cautiously.
2. Breathe normally.

Next the 'Don'ts':
1. No jerks.
2. No strain.
3. Pregnant women must avoid this asana.

## What good is this Asana to us ?

1. It increases flexibility of the spine.
2. Cures constipation and dyspepsia.
3. Benefits the thyroid and parathyroid glands
4. Regulates metabolism, and
5. A sure remedy for a flabby abdomen.

# BHUJANGASANA

**This has something to do with cobra, isn't it ?**

Indeed, it's the cobra pose. The cobra is a snake and the snake is also called 'sarpa' and so this pose is often called Sarpasana. But, the Sanskrit word for snake is 'Bhujanga'. Therefore, this asana is known by the term Bhujangasana.

**I find from the illustration that we begin by lying flat on the abdomen, with legs and feet together and soles turned up.**

Yes, and if you see the illustration carefully you'll find that the hands are placed by the side of the chest with elbows bent, and the tips of the fingers are in line with the shoulders and the forehead touching the ground.

**Then, what ?**

Follow these stages...

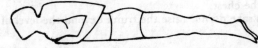

*Stage 1:* Push your nose forward slightly till it brushes against the floor and move the chin forward.

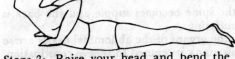

*Stage 2:* Raise your head and bend the neck backwards compressing the nape but take care to keep your chest close to the ground.

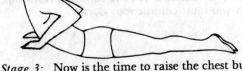

*Stage 3:* Now is the time to raise the chest but try to do this without the help of the arms and turn the eyes to the ceiling.

## What is the objective here ?

The objective here is to let the pressure in the spine travel down from the neck region to the middle of the back.

## Then what about the arms ?

Yes, once you have raised your chest, you can take the help of the arms to raise your back further so that the lower part of the back too is raised.

In this pose, you'll see that finally the spine forms a deep curve.

Reverse the order and you are where you started from.

## Are there any special points to remember ?

Concentrate on the spinal column as a whole.

In the beginning, you may find it difficult to raise your chest without the help of your arms, in which case the arms may be used.

Take care to see that the elbows are not spread. Hold them near the chest.

For God's sake do *not* raise the trunk beyond the level of the navel.

## The advantages are obvious—aren't they ? It is the spine that benefits, isn't it ?

Yes, indeed, the spine becomes supple and the back is prevented from suffering.

What is more, the organs of the abdominal cavity are so toned up that this asana is reputed to relieve constipation, rid you of your flatulence, and even correct the irregularities of the menstrual cycle.

And lastly, it also gives relief to certain types of slipped disc problem but, of course, if you are suffering from this, before you start you must consult your doctor.

# ARDHA SHALABHASANA

**What does this pose signify ?**

It is half-locust pose.

**Why is it compared to a locust or a half locust ?**

In this pose you raise one leg at a time like the hind part of a locust. Hence it is called Ardha Shalabhasana.

**Can you enumerate the technique ?**

Yes, it is as follows:

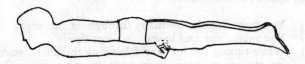

*Stage 1:*
You lie flat, but on your abdomen and then,
(a) keep your feet together,
(b) point the toes backward,
(c) place the arms extended on the sides with closed fingers,
(d) place the knuckles on the ground,
(e) rest the chin on the floor,
(f) stretch the neck, and
(g) thus compress the nape.

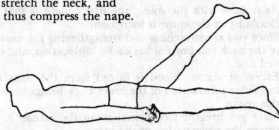

*Stage 2:*
Raise your right leg slowly as much as you can without bending it at the knee and maintain the pose comfortably for sometime.

*Stage 3:*
Lower the leg slowly to stage 1.

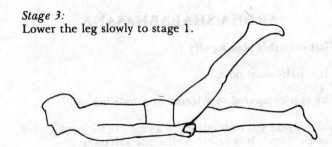

*Stage 4:*
Repeat stages 2 and 3 with the left leg.

**Any special instructions ?**

(1)   You must breathe normally throughout the asana.
(2)   You must raise and lower your legs slowly.
(3)   While raising the legs avoid bending the knees, making the calves tense, or putting any pressure on the other knee.

It must be noted here that once you have learnt this pose, viz. Ardha Shalabhasana, you are ready for the full asana viz. Shalabhasana.

**I suppose there are specific beneficial effects of this pose.**

Naturally!

1.   As it deals with the spine, the first benefit is that the flexibility of the spine is increased.
2.   Since you are stretching and strengthening the muscles of the back you prevent backache, dislocation, and slipped disc.
3.   Excess of venous blood is forced from the veins and muscular contraction of the lower back brings blood to this region.
4.   Since you breathe freely throughout the asana, it improves the oxygenation of the lungs.
5.   Since you increase the pressure in the abdominal viscera, the functions of the liver, the pancreas, and the intestines are improved.

# SHALABHASANA

**Oh! This is the full asana of the half locust pose you were talking of, isn't it?**

Yes, it is, and since you have learnt the Ardha Shalabhasana you are now ready for the full asana.

**Is the technique the same ?**

Yes, in so far as the starting position is concerned. However, in this pose —

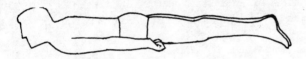

*Stage 1 :* You inhale a little.

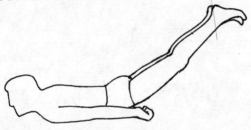

*Stage 2 :* Pressing on the wrists, you raise both your legs as much as you can without bending, and then,
*Stage 3:* Slowly bring down the legs, and
*Stage 4:* Exhale.

**I suppose the cautions are the same as in Ardha Shalabhasana, are they ?**

Yes, except that here you have to be extra careful. While keeping the fists close to your body and the knuckles down, you may find some difficulty in raising both the legs.

## In that case how does one overcome this difficulty ?

The way out is to keep your fists under the thighs, so that the legs can be raised easily. And, of course, remember the following:
1. No jerks in raising the legs,
2. No bending of knees,
3. Nor of elbows either.

## Are the advantages double ?

Yes, indeed, but there are also dangers in this asana for those suffering from heart and lung diseases and even diseases of the abdominal organs.

# DHANURASANA

**In this picture the body appears like a bow ?**

Yes, the backward curl of the body resembles a bow. 'Dhanu' in Sanskrit means the 'bow' and this asana is formed by the bending of the body while the hands and the legs form the string of the bow.

**But we have had similar asanas before, haven't we ?**

Yes, we have. Actually this is a combination of two asanas about which you know something already, viz. Bhujangasana and Shalabhasana.

**But how do we start this asana and what are the stages ?**

You lie on your stomach, with arms on the side and your back fully relaxed.

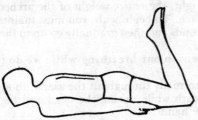

*Stage 1* :  You bend your legs at the knee joints till they are folded upon the thighs.

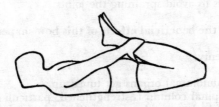

*Stage 2* :  You catch the right ankle with the right hand, and the left one with the left hand.

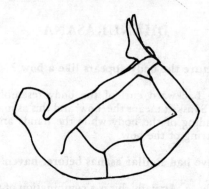

*Stage 3* :  Tugging at the legs firmly you try to arch the body
          backward, by raising the head, the body, and the
          knees.

**Yes, the picture shows the whole arched body on the
stomach, doesn't it ?**

  You are right, the entire weight of the arched body rests
on the stomach. To begin with, you must maintain the pose
for a few seconds and then gradually go up to three minutes.

**What happens to our breathing while we do this asana ?**

  Breathe normally throughout the asana, though you may
hold the breath while raising the head and tugging at the
legs with the hands.

*Caution*

  Utmost care must be taken not to perform this asana in
jerks, so as to avoid spraining the joints.

**What are the beneficial effects of this bow shaped asana ?**

  Oh ! plenty.

1.  The abdominal organs get toned up.
2.  The spinal column is strengthened, particularly at the
    cervical, thoracic, lumbar, and sacral regions, i.e., the
    last four bones of the spine.

## Any glandular stimulation ?

That's a good question. This asana stimulates the endocrine glands, i.e., the suprarenal, thyroid glands, and because there is a lot of intra-abdominal pressure, the digestive system is toned up effectively.

# VAKRASANA

**This pose is evidently meant for the waist, isn't that so?**

Yes, it is known as the twist-pose where we practise a twist of the trunk, and since the Sanskrit word for twist is 'Vakra' the pose is called Vakrasana.

**Is it a sitting pose?**

Yes, you start by sitting with legs extended.

**Are there many stages?**

Yes, quite a few. These are:

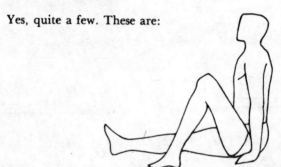

*Stage 1* : You bend your left leg at the knee and place it near the right knee.

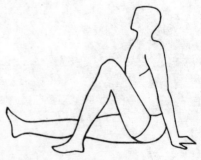

*Stage 2* : Place your left hand at the back in line with the spine and sit erect.

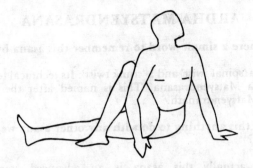

*Stage 3* : Bring your right hand over the left knee and place it on the left side.

*Stage 4* : Press the raised knee with the right upper arm and twist the trunk to the left. Look as far back as possible.

*Stage 5* : Release the twist.

*Stage 6* : Withdraw the crossed right hand and place it on the right side.

*Stage 7* : Remove the left hand placed at the back and bring it on the left side.

*Stage 8* : Extend the left leg.

Repeat the same procedure on the other side, giving right twist to the spine.

## Any special method to follow while twisting?

The correct way to twist the body is to press the knee firmly with the elbow.

## And the benefits are to the waist?

To the spine, to be more precise. This asana makes the spine flexible. And what's move, the pressure exerted on the abdominal viscera improves the function of the abdominal organs.

# ARDHA MATSYENDRASANA

**Isn't there a simple word to remember this asana by ?**

It is a 'spinal twist' and a 'trunk twist'. Its technical term is Sulabha Matsyendrasana. This is named after the great Yogi, Matsyendranath.

**Hasn't this anything to do with any other asana we have learnt ?**

Yes, actually this asana is an advanced stage of Vakrasana. Here you start with the legs extended. The stages are:

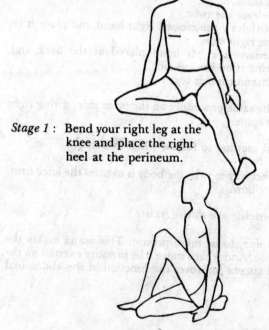

*Stage 1 :* Bend your right leg at the knee and place the right heel at the perineum.

*Stage 2 :* Bend the left leg, but see that the left foot is placed on the outer side of the right thigh.

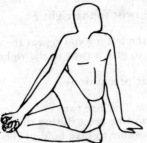

## And then ?

Then comes *stage 3*, when you turn the trunk to the left, cross the right arm over the left knee and catch hold of the left big toe with the right hand.

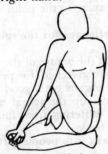

*Stage 4* : Now turn the trunk a little more to the left, with the chin over the left shoulder. Take the left hand over the back, and get a firm hold of the right thigh.

*Stage 5* : Now twist the spine, but steadily, keeping the chest erect and forward.

*Stage 6* : Maintain the pose as long as you comfortably can for about five seconds to begin with.

## Now the unwinding ?

Yes, but steadily and stage by stage.
— First, release the hold on the right thigh and remove the twist of the spine.
— Next, release the hold on the left foot and place the right hand on the side.
— Extend the left and then the right leg, and back to the starting position.

**What about the twist to the right ?**

Starting with the left leg you repeat the entire procedure in a reverse way to give a twist to the right side.

**What about your precautions ?**

Yes, among the 'Dos' are two:
(1) The trunk must be erect during the twist, and
(2) If it is not possible to take hold of the thigh, place the hand on the ground in order to get a good twist.

As for the 'Don'ts', only one is important:
Do not twist the spine to the point of discomfort.

**I suppose the benefits are for the spine ?**

Yes, the spine and the organs of the pelvic region. Firstly, the pelvic muscles are stretched, the pelvic joints made flexible, and the pelvic organs get a good circulation of blood. The asana also tones up the spinal nerves. Secondly, this asana helps people suffering from *lumbago* and muscular rheumatism in the back.

But the best benefit is to people suffering from constipation.

# PADAHASTASANA

**This is one of those poses we were taught in our school. They used to tell us it makes our body flexible. Is this true?**

Very true. It is called Padahastasana, since 'Pada' means feet and 'Hasta' means hands. Obviously, the very name suggests that it's a pose where the hands are brought closer to the feet.

**Is it just standing erect and attempting to touch our feet?**

**Yes, but there are stages:**

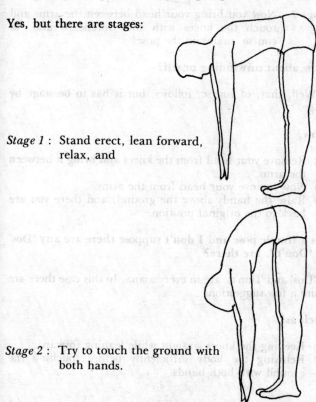

*Stage 1* :  Stand erect, lean forward, relax, and

*Stage 2* :  Try to touch the ground with both hands.

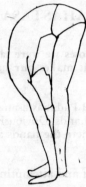

*Stage 3* : Now you bring your head between the arms and touch the knees with your forehead, and, of course, maintain the pose.

**How about unwinding onself?**

Well, that, of course, follows, but it has to be stage by stage.

**How?**

(1) Remove your head from the knees and bring it between the arms.
(2) Now remove your head from the arms.
(3) Raise the hands above the ground, and there you are back to the original position.

**It's a simple pose and I don't suppose there are any 'Dos' or 'Don'ts', are there?**

'Dos' and 'Don'ts' are in every asana. In this case there are quite a few suggestions.

**Such as?**

(1) Keeping the knees straight while leaning forward.
(2) Relaxing the body sufficiently before touching the ground with both hands.

(3) Keeping the feet apart perhaps in the beginning, and
    later keeping them together.

    And, of course, all this has to be done without jerks,
    particularly while leaning forward and later returning
    to the standing position.

(4) Exhale while leaning forward to facilitate better flexion.

**And all this makes the body flexible, does it?**

Yes, Sir, it does make the body flexible by stretching the
back and hamstring muscles.

Actually this asana leads to another one, viz.
'Paschimatanasana'.

# PASCHIMATANASANA OR
# PASCHIMOTTANASANA

**This is too big a word, can you explain it ?**

'Paschima' in Sanskrit means 'posterior', while 'tana' means 'stretch'. Since in this pose you stretch your back or the posterior part of your body, you call this important asana, the Paschimatanasana.

**Is the technique the usual one, i.e. starting with the legs extended and together ?**

Yes, and the stages that follow are:

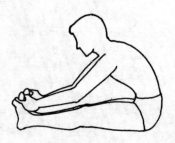

*Stage 1* : Bend your index fingers to form a hook and hold the great toes with them and bend the elbows.

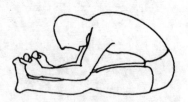

*Stage 2* : Exhale while bending forward, bringing your head between the hands.

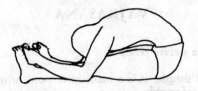

*Stage 3* : Bending the elbows and the trunk further, try to touch the knees with your forehead — without raising the knees, mind you !

*Stage 4* : Inhale now, as you raise your head slowly bringing it between the hands.

*Stage 5* : Raise the trunk and the head leaving the toes and straightening the spine — and with your hands on the sides you are back to the starting position.

## What about your cautions and precautions ?

(1) If you want anything to facilitate bending, it is exhaling when bending.

(2) Bend as far as you comfortably can and maintain the position in a relaxed manner. In other words, don't strain while bending.

(3) But, for God's sake, don't bend forward or return in a jerky manner.

(4) Again, while touching the knees don't raise them from the ground.

(5) Beware ! If you are a *slipped disc* patient or are suffering from *spondylosis,* you must do this asana only under expert supervision.

## What are the regions that get the benefits, if any ?

Firstly, this asana gives a steady stretch to the back and thigh muscles, and makes the spine flexible and elastic. Secondly, the abdomen and the abdominal organs are affected the most and, therefore, the digestive system is toned up, and bowel movement is helped.

# VAJRASANA

**Is this also a pelvic pose?**

Plain and simple, it is a meditative pose, which you can maintain comfortably.

**I suppose the start is the usual one: We sit with legs extended and together, correct?**

Correct.

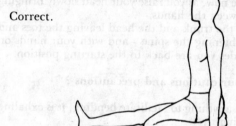

*Stage 1* : Bending it at the knee, the left leg is folded upon itself. You turn it back and place the sole under

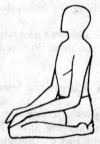

the buttock, with toes pointing inward.

*Stage 2* : The right sole is similarly arranged under the right buttock.

*Stage 3* : With palm on the knees and the knees close together, sit comfortably.

*Stage 4* : Keep the spine erect, eyes closed, the body relaxed, and concentrate on breathing and there you have your meditative pose.

Here are a few 'Dos' — not many, only three.
1.   Draw the heels out of the buttocks.
2.   Keep the trunk and the head erect.
3.   Sit in the asana as long as it is comfortable.

Remember only one 'Don't' — Don't sit on the heels.

## What about the advantages?

The fact that it is a comfortable sitting position is itself an advantage. The other advantages are that it exercises the thigh muscles and prevents stiff knees and ankle joints.

# SUPTAVAJRASANA

**Here we don't begin by lying on our back, do we?**

No, You begin by sitting with your legs extended.

**And then?**

And then —

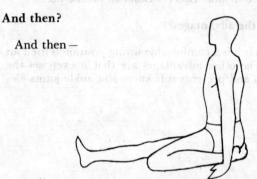

*Stage 1* : You bend the left leg at the knee, turn it backward and place it on the left side near the buttocks.

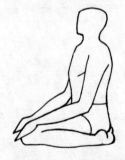

*Stage 2* : Next you do the same with the right leg.

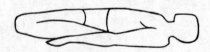

*Stage 3* : Now taking support of the elbows, you try to lie on the back.

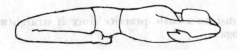

*Stage 4* : As for the arms, holding the opposite shoulders you keep the arms under the head.

*Stage 5* : Leaving the grasp of the shoulders, you now sit up in Vajrasana, taking the help of the elbows.

*Stage 6* : And back to normal by extending the right and left legs in turn.

**Isn't this a difficult pose with the legs turned backward at the knees and also lying on the back?**

Perhaps yes, but in the beginning you keep your knees apart while lying on the back and only by gradual stages do you bring them together and, of course, you reduce the arch at the lumbar region very gradually and avoid dropping the body in a jerky manner during the backward movement.

**I suppose the asana obviously benefits the spine, doesn't it?**

Well said, indeed. A steady stretch to the vertebrae and muscles of the lumbar region, and the stretch to the abdominal region give proper stimuli to the abdominal organs and thus helps move the bowels regularly.

# YOGAMUDRA

**This must be a basic practice since it straightway deals with yoga.**

   Correct, the synonym for this practice is
— Yoga lock
— Cross-legged forward bend
In fact, it is a lotus position with forward bending.

**How does one perform this practise ?**

   Starting position: Sit with legs extended.

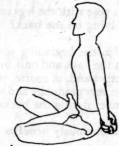

*Stage 1 :* Sit in Padmasana.
*Stage 2 :* Hold your hands at the back catching the right wrist with the left hand.

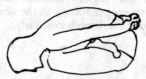

*Stage 3 :* Now slowly bend the trunk forward and touch the ground with the forehead.

**How long do we maintain this position ?**

*Stage 4 :* Maintain this pose for a comfortable time (breathing normally) while relaxing the muscles which are not in action.

**What happens next ?**

*Stage 5* : Raise the trunk slowly and release the hold of your hands.

*Stage 6* : You lift the left foot with your hands and extend it.

*Stage 7* : Then you extend the right foot and assume the starting position.

## Are any precautions necessary ?

Yes, there are

1. For instance, keep the two heels quite close to the abdomen .
2. The trunk must be bent and raised slowly, and remember not to strain in the beginning when you desire to touch the ground with your forehead.

## Is that easy ?

Easy, of course but only after sufficient practice.

## How about summing up the advantages ?

Advantage 1: General tone up of the abdominal organs.
Advantage 2: Constipation is prevented, and this posture makes the spine flexible.

# PARVATASANA

This word too is easy to understand. It's based on 'par-vata' which we ordinarily use for 'mountain', isn't that so?

Yes, in this pose you put your hands in the shape of a cone, and this conical shape formed by the hands looks like the peak of a 'paravata' (mountain).

**How does one go about it ? I suppose we begin by the usual 'Padmasana'.**

Yes, you seem to get the hang of it, don't you ? But remember, instead of Padmasana, any other comfortable position would do.

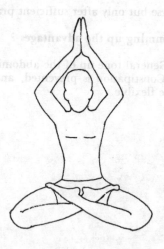

*Stage 1 :* You raise both your hands sideward and join them over the head, at the same time inhaling. I mean simultaneously.

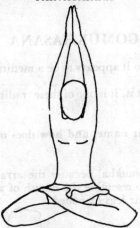

*Stage 2 :* You further inhale deeply and stretch your hands as high as possible. While maintaining this position you continue your normal breathing.

*Stage 3 :* While exhaling lower the hands over your head.

*Stage 4 :* Then bring the hands down on the sides, exhaling simultaneously.

## But where should we put the hands before and after raising them ?

They must be placed on the knees and remember to maintain the position of the hands over the head for just a few seconds.

## Will you tell us the important 'Dos' and 'Dont s' and the beneficial effects ?

(1) Let your body be erect, in other words, don't bend forward or backward.

(2) You do use your neck in this asana and so your neck and back are also stengthened.

(3) Obviously this asana keeps .the arthritis of the shoulders away.

(4) Since the muscles of your ribs get an exercise, they too become more flexible.

(5) This asana also relieves tension in the neck and shoulder muscles.

# GOMUKHASANA

**From the diagram it appears to be a meditative pose. Is it?**

You are right, it is. It is one of these traditional meditative poses.

**Why this peculiar name, and how does one practise this asana?**

It is called 'Gomukha' because the arrangement of the legs is supposed to resemble the mouth of a cow.
You sit with your legs extended—

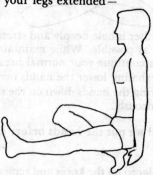

*Stage 1:* Bend the right leg at the knee and place the heel on the left side close to the buttocks.

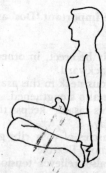

*Stage 2:* Do the same with the left leg, finally bringing the knees one over the other.

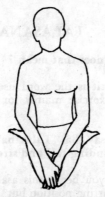

*Stage 3*    Sit erect, with your hands on the knees, and
maintaining the meditative pose, breathe normally. And now unwind yourself, as it were.

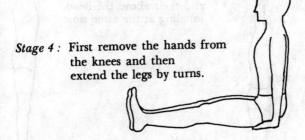

*Stage 4 :*    First remove the hands from
the knees and then
extend the legs by turns.

## What about your hints ?

(1) Press the heels against the buttocks,
(2) Sit erect without bending at the loins, and
(3) Keep the knees one over the other.

    Remember, you are not to sit on your heels.

    This asana may be practised by changing the positions of
the legs and the hands.

    And the main benefit you get from this asana is that it
gives you the flexibility of the hip joints.

# TALASANA

**Talasana—What does that mean ?**

'Tala' in Sanskrit is the word used for the palm tree. Talasana is an exercise mainly for stretching the whole body.

**Would you then say that 'Talasana' is a posture like the palm tree and standing tall and stretching ?**

It is true that you begin this asana standing with feet together as the starting position but, while you stand erect, the body must feel relaxed. Now follow these stages:

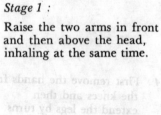

*Stage 1 :*

Raise the two arms in front and then above the head, inhaling at the same time.

*Stage 2 :* Raise the heels and balance on the toes. (After learning the asana Stages 1 and 2 can be done simultaneously).

*Stage 3 :* Now is the time to pose like a spread out palm tree. So you give an extra stretch upward with a little more inhalation, holding out for a few seconds. And then the reverse—

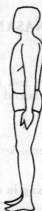

*Stages 4:* Heels down, bring the arms down from the front
&5   while exhaling gradually, thus coming back to the
     original position. And now for the usual instruc-
     tions.

Start with your feet a little apart till you get your balance.
Later on, with a little practice you can keep the feet
together. But take care not to bend either at the waist or at
the knees.

## Of what particular good is this asana, and why ?

Why not examine the very act of this asana, shall we ?

1. In this asana, where does the weight of your body fall? It
   falls on the front part of the legs, which means it gives
   strength to your ankle joints.
2. Normally in our daily routine we hardly exercise our
   chest and back muscles, but when we perform this asana,
   we exercise them sufficiently.
3. Further, with this asana the chances of getting a slipped
   disc are remote. This asana stretches the spine, and
   perhaps it is reasonable to claim that it improves the
   height.
4. Do this asana, and you prevent arthritis of the shoulder
   joints, and
5. Finally, your breathing system naturally becomes more
   efficient.

# KONASANA

**What does 'Kona' mean?**

'Kona' means an angle, and so Konasana stands for 'Angular' posture and also lateral stretch.

**Do we stand or sit?**

Stand—and that too erect—keeping your feet about 60 cms apart.

**I suppose we do so breathing in and out—Don't we?**

My friend, all yogic asanas are accompanied by appropriate type of breathing.

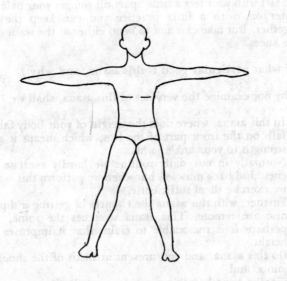

*Stage 1:* For instance in this asana you breathe in and stretch your hands out.

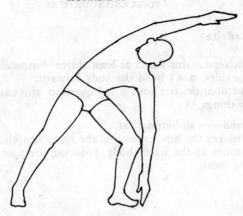

*Stage 2:* Bend at the left knee and slide the left arm down the left leg to touch the ground. Simultaneously raise the right arm up.

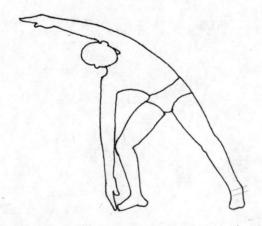

*Stage 3:* Now you breathe out and return to stage 1.

*Stage 4:* Bend at the right knee and slide the right arm down the right leg to touch the ground and raise the left arm simultaneously.

*Stage 5:* Breathe out and return to the starting position.

**Any advice?**

Yes, repeat this asana at least thrice, but while bending on the sides, *don't* bend the body forward.

And to anticipate your usual question, this exercise does many things:

1. It reduces abdominal fat.
2. It makes the hip region and the spine flexible, and
3. It tones up the whole body, reducing the pain, if any in the loins.

# TRIKONASANA

**What does this word mean?**

In Sanskrit 'trikona' means a triangle.

**But what are the three sides of this triangle?**

That's a good question. In this posture the arm, the leg and the trunk form a triangle.

**Do we start sitting comfortably or standing erect?**

In this asana you begin by standing with your feet approximately 60 cms. apart.

**What about the position of the arms?**

The arms are by the sides.

**Can you tell us the different stages?**

Yes, the stages are:

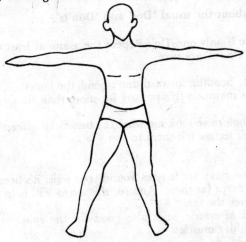

*Stage 1:* While breathing in, raise your arms sidewards and keep the feet approximately 60 cms apart.

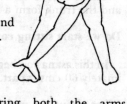

*Stage 2:*  While breathing out, bend your body
            forward and touch the right toes
            with the fingers of your left hand.

*Stage 3:*  Raise your right arm up and
            look up at the right hand.

*Stage 4:*  While breathing in bring both the arms
            sidewards.

*Stage 5:*  While breathing out, bring the arms to the
            original position.

Repeat the asana on the other side.

## What about the usual 'Dos' and 'Don'ts'?

There is only one 'Do': Repeat the asana at least thrice.
The 'Don'ts' are two:

1. While bending forward don't bend the knees.
2. Don't maintain this posture for more than six seconds.

And before you ask me what the beneficial effects of this
pose are, let *me* tell them to you.

1.  If you have 'spare tyres' round your waist it's because of
    the extra fat there. And so, this asana will help you to
    reduce the fat.
2.  And of course, it is also good for the spine and the
    shoulder muscles.

# CHAKRASANA

**Do we in this asana form a 'Chakra' or a wheel?**

Almost so. As the form of this pose resembles a circle, we call it Chakrasana.

**Does this start with the usual 'Padmasana'?**

Oh, no! Here you stand with your feet together and the stages are:

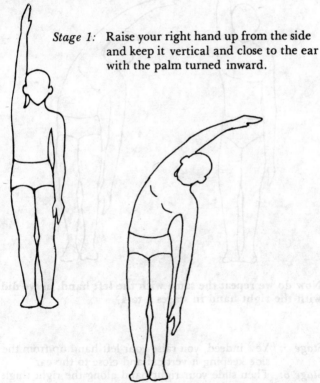

*Stage 1:*   Raise your right hand up from the side and keep it vertical and close to the ear with the palm turned inward.

*Stage 2:*   Slide your hand along the left thigh up to the knee and bend your body on the left side as much as possible.

*Stages 3*
*& 4:*          Slide the left hand upward and assume the erect
               position, and then bring the right hand down
               from the side.

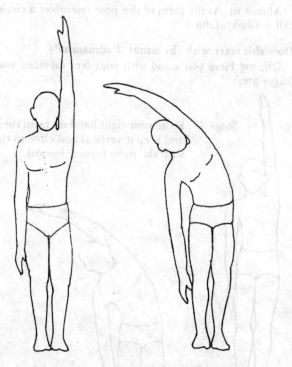

**Now do we repeat the same with the left hand, as we did
with the right hand in stages 1 to 4?**

*Stage 5:*   Yes, indeed, you raise your left hand up from the
             side keeping it vertical and close to the ear.
*Stage 6:*   Then slide your right hand along the right thigh
             as in stage 2, and so on till you do the same and
             end up as in stage 4, where you will have the left
             hand down from the side.

## What are the special precautions in this asana?

They are the usual 'Do s' such as:
1. Go slow—no jerky or fast movements, and
2. Keep your body erect, i.e. there should be no bending forward or backward.

## And the beneficial effects?

Since you do a lot of bending laterally it helps the spine to be flexible.

There is considerable movement of the ribs as well as the muscles of the loins and so, this helps to relieve aches. Finally, remember, for full benefit, this asana should be repeated several times.

# KANTHASANA

**Are there any asanas for the neck ?**

Yes, there are. One of them is called Kanthasana or Brahma Mudra.

**What is the purpose of these asanas ?**

They are meant to provide exercise to the neck muscles as also to the cervical spine.

**What is the technique of Kanthasana?**

The simplest one can think of. All that you do is:

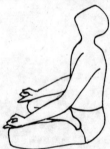

1. Bend the head as far *back* as possible but at the same time you *breathe in* and then slowly bring it back to its original position while breathing out.

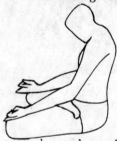

2. In the same way you lower the neck breathing out of course, and then bring it back to its original position while breathing in.

**Are there any left and right movements also ?**

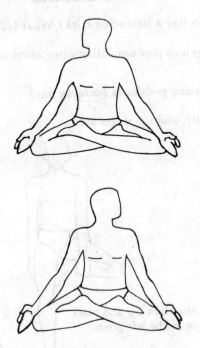

Obviously, now you turn your head to *the right* while breathing in, and back again to the *original* position while breathing out. Next, you turn your head to the left, breathing in, and back to the original postion, breathing out at the same time. Remember, all the movements should be done slowly.

**Any curative aspect of this asana ?**

Yes, it is beneficial in cases of spondylosis, stiff neck, and frozen shoulders.

# VRIKSHASANA

**This looks like a balancing trick? What is it?**

Actually it's a pose simulating a tree where you balance on your leg.

**Is the starting position a standing one?**

Naturally, and the stages are:

1. Raise the right leg and place the foot in the left groin.

2. Place folded hands on the chest.

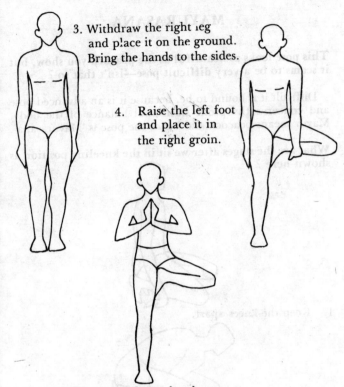

3. Withdraw the right leg and place it on the ground. Bring the hands to the sides.

4. Raise the left foot and place it in the right groin.

5. Place folded hands on the chest.
6. Withdraw the left leg and place it on the ground. Bring the hands to the sides.

## Any hint?

Yes. In the beginning you may make use of your hands—though only in the beginning—to place your feet on the groins by turns.

## Any caution?

People who have balancing difficulties or problems with their balancing mechanism should consult their doctor before practising this asana.

# MAYURASANA

This pose looks as beautiful as the peacock you show, but it seems to be a very difficult pose—isn't that so ?

Difficult it is bound to be, because it is an advanced pose and concerns the prone horizontal balance of the body. Mayur means peacock and hence the pose is 'Mayurasana'.

What are the stages after we sit in the kneeling position as shown here ?

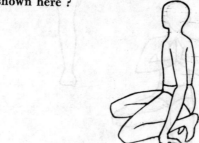

1. Keep the knees apart.

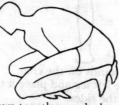

2. Place both elbows together and place the hands on the ground, fingers pointing backwards towards the toes.

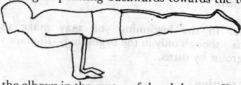

3. Place the elbows in the centre of the abdomen. Keep the hands firm and, supporting the whole body against the elbows, stretch out the legs.

4. Inhale and lift the legs slowly to a level with the head and balance the body horizontal with the ground.

**Maintaining this position must be really difficult. What does one do after that ?**

5. Bring the legs to the ground.
6. Bringing the legs closer, touch the knees to the ground.
7. Remove the hands and place them on the sides.
8. Reduce the distance between the knees and return to the starting position.

**There must be some 'Dos' and 'Don'ts'—aren't there any?**

Yes, they are in the form of suggestions:

1. Move the body forward and then raise the legs slowly while maintaining the balance.
2. To get a firm hold of the ground, it's a useful hint to spread your fingers like the toes of a peacock.
3. Don't let your knees bend, and don't droop your chin. Remember, you are to be 'as proud as the peacock', and so 'chin up, brudder !'.
4. Remember, no *jerks* at all !

**And the benefits ?**

These are obvious. You improve your poise and balance. The pressure on the stomach improves blood circulation.

*Caution:*

Fatty people, particularly women with weak arms and loose abdomen, are advised to avoid this pose.

# PAVANA MUKTASANA

### Is there any asana that relieves us of gas ?

The asana that is useful for this purpose is called 'Pavan-muktasana'. 'Pavana' means wind and mukta 'means' release.

### How do we manage it ?

By following these stages:

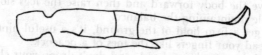

1.  You lie supine, i.e. face upward,

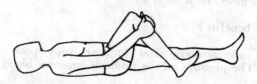

2.  Next you raise one leg and bend it at the knee and try to press the bent leg firmly on the abdomen, with both the hands.

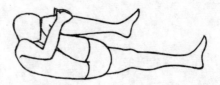

3.  Now try to touch the knee with your head keeping the other leg extended without bending it, and then do the same with the other leg.

## Why do we use only one leg ?

Well, you may use both the legs too.

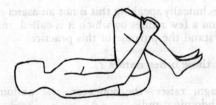

1. Bend them at the knees.
2. Keep them a little apart, hold them between the arms and press them firmly against the abdomen.

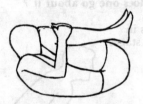

3. Again try to touch the knees with your forehead.
4. Maintain this pose comfortably.
5. Now try to contract and release alternately, your anus or what they strictly call anal *sphincters*, the last few muscular rings on the lowest end of your food canal.

## The main advantage is the expulsion of gas—Isn't it so ?

Of course, it does help expulsion of gas but the fact that you use your legs and the stomach and the arms—all go to tone up several muscles like:

(a) those of the back,
(b) those of the lumbar region,
(c) those of the abdomen,
     and above all, it helps bowel movement.

# UDDIYANA BANDHA

**What on earth is this asana or posture for ?**

Well, technically speaking this is not an asana or posture. If I give you a few names by which it is called, may be, you will understand the purpose of this practice.

**What are those other names ?**

Diaphragm raiser—the squeezer—the abdominal lock and the abdominal pull.

**Yes, the names are suggestive, for they make one thing clear, viz. the practice has to do a lot with the abdomen. Anyway, how does one go about it ?**

The answer is in
the following stages:

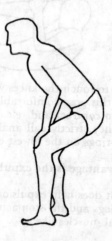

*Stage 1* :  Stand straight with your feet 30-45 cms apart.
*Stage 2* :  Bend your trunk forward and your knees too a little.
*Stage 3* :  Your palms are on your thighs.
*Stage 4* :  Contract vigorously your abdominal muscles and breathe out completely, as if you are emptying your lungs.

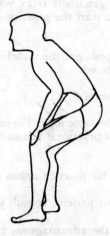

*Stage 5* : Now relax slowly the abdominal muscles which you had contracted in stage 4.

*Stage 6* : Simultaneously hold the breath and imitate the movement of deep inspiration trying to expand the rib cage.

*Stage 7* : You will feel your diaphragm move up and your abdomen will cave in and look hollow. Hold the breath for a few seconds.

*Stage 8* : By now you will start feeling uncomfortable. That is the signal to relax and allow the thoracic or rib cage to become normal.

## Any 'Dos' and 'Don'ts' ?

Of course, if you think carefully, these 'Dos' and 'Don'ts' will work themselves out.

For instance, this Yogic exercise has to do with the movement of the abdomen; so, it's commonsense that you keep your stomach empty, isn't it ?

1. Well then, here is the first 'Do'. Keep your stomach empty.
2. You must exhale or breathe out fully i.e. the lungs must remain empty.

Then, unless you genuinely relax your abdominal wall muscles how can you start the practice ? And so, the third 'Do' is :

3.  In the starting position, the muscles of the abdominal wall must be relaxed.

**What about the 'Don'ts' ?**

You get them by the same logic. For instance, it's impossible for you to do this practice if you suffer from abdominal pain.

1.  So, don't start this practice unless you have consulted your doctor.
2.  If you are a heart patient, consult your doctor.

**Tell me, what are the advantageous effects of this practice?**

With this practice it is natural to expect improvement in abdominal circulation and you don't get either indigestion or constipation. And don't forget, with the abdomen, organs like the liver, the pancreas, and the spleen also get good blood circulation. This practice also stimulates the lungs.

**But why these three organs particularly?**

If you look at the location, they are under your diaphragm. You already know that in this particular practice which is a diaphragm raiser, blood flows freely through these organs. Then, need I tell you that this practice also stimulates the lungs?

**Is this the only practice that can claim to be the corrective for abdominal troubles?**

No, I believe there is another practice known as 'Nauli' which is more effective. But we are not considering it for the present.

# TADAGI MUDRA

**Has this practice anything to do with the stomach ?**

You have guessed that correctly. In fact, 'abdominal depression' is another way of naming this practice.

**Hasn't this practice a similarity with another practice ?**

Another correct guess. The Uddiyana Bandha which is described earlier, is very similar to this one. Anyway, here's what you do in this practice. Of course, you begin as usual, lying supine i.e. with face upwards.

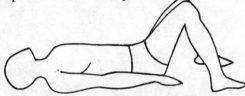

*Stage 1 :* Draw the feet closer, keeping the knees raised up.

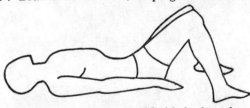

*Stage 2 :* Exhale completely, and hold the breath.
*Stage 3 :* Holding the breath and not allowing air to enter the lung, expand the chest.
*Stage 4 :* After a few seconds lower the ribs, and
*Stage 5 :* Inhale.

**What if we cannot control the passage of air into the lungs while expanding the chest ?**

In such a case close your nose and mouth in the beginning and relax the abdominal muscles. Remember to avoid holding the breath for more than 5 seconds, in the beginning.

## What are the beneficial effects ?

The same as those in Uddiyana. By the creation of negative pressure in the abdomen, blood circulation is *promoted* and very naturally the functions of the abdominal organs improve.

## Any precautions ?

Yes, those who have a weak heart or circulatory abnormalities, must not perform this practice except with the guidance of a yoga expert and under medical advice.

# AGNISARA

**The word leads me to believe this practice has something to do with 'fire'. Is that right?**

Yes, this practice stimulates what we call 'gastric fire'. Actually it's the abdominal press and push.

**Of what use is this practice ?**

Talking of benefits straightaway, it is one of the cleansing processes.

**What are its stages ?**

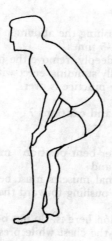

*Stage 1* : Stand erect, with the feet apart.
*Stage 2* : Bend forward, place the hands on the knees, exhale fully, and hold the breath.

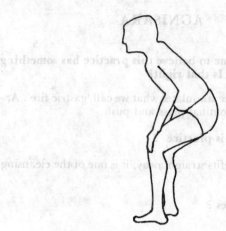

*Stage 3* :  Start pushing the abdomen in and out vigorously about 4-5 times.

*Stage 4* :  Inhale deeply, remove the hands from the knees, gradually standing erect with your feet together, and the practice is over.

**Any suggestions and cautions ?**

Yes,

1. The shoulder-bent-position must be **maintained** throughout, and
2. The abdominal muscles must be kept stiff while contracting and pushing forward the abdomen.

The only caution here is, do not be tempted to raise the ribs and expand the chest while pressing the abdomen inward.

As for the advantages, it's obvious the abdomen and the abdominal organs take the largest measure of benefits.

*Important:* Will those of you who suffer from hyperacidity, or ulcer, and tenderness in the abdomen, please keep away from this practice ?

# SHAVASANA

### Is it the pose where you look like a dead body?

Very true. This is the corpse like pose. In this posture you completely relax the body as if it is dead and the mind too has to be emptied of thoughts.

### How can one relax the mind?

By keeping the body motionless and then attempting to drive away all thoughts, from your mind. You see, the word 'Shava' means in Sanskrit a dead body and a dead body presupposes a dead mind, too. This asana does appear easy, but complete supine relaxation requires a technique.

### Let's know the technique.

Watch these stages:

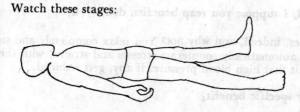

*Stage 1:* Lie flat—limbs, too, in a relaxed position—upper limbs making an angle of 15 degrees with the trunk and the lower ones about 30 degrees apart.

### What about the forearms and fingers?

They too must be in a comfortable position with the fingers semiflexed.

*Stage 2:* Close the eyes with drooping eyelids, breathing deeply yes, unusually deeper and longer. Of course, your abdomen will make free movements—bulging out while breathing in and going in while breathing out.

**How long does one do that?**

Well, the job is to concentrate on this abdominal move-ment, and it will take you about 2 weeks to establish this rhythm. And now begin the fine points in *stage 3* which is concentration on (1) the sensation at the nostrils, (2) the *coolness* of the inspired air, and (3) the warmth of the ex-pired air. Remember, when you concentrate on breathing—particularly these fine aspects of the asana, the muscles of your body will automatically relax further.

**I suppose there are things you should do and those that you shouldn't?**

No, not many except that whilst relaxing you maintain your body in a position once taken, and you will make no movements except breathing as explained above.

**And, I suppose you reap benefits, don't you?**

Yes, indeed, and why not? You relax completely and so you automatically counteract stresses and strains, with the result that high blood pressure, if any, gets reduced.

**Any specific benefit?**

Yes, migraine and any other stress-related disorders disappear and hot conditions also improve. It particularly helps in reducing high blood pressure.

# MAKARASANA

**What is this pose for ?**

It's a relaxing posture like the Shavasana, but in the prone position. It resembles a crocodile which generally appears relaxed.

**How does one secure this pose ?**

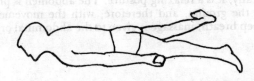

*Stage 1* : By lying in the prone position, keeping a distance of about 20-30 cms between the feet.
*Stage 2* : By placing the ankles on the ground and heels on the inner side touching the ground.

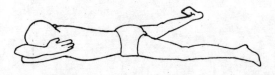

*Stage 3* : By holding the right shoulder with the left hand and similarly the left shoulder with the right hand.
*Stage 4* : By placing the forehead between the arms and relaxing completely.

**How long does one maintain this pose ?**

About 2 or 3 minutes, before unwinding yourself as it were.

**Suggestions ?**

Only a few.
1.  Spread the legs in such a manner that the pelvic region is firmly pressed to the ground.
2.  While placing the head between the arms, make certain that you are able to breathe comfortably.
3.  The chest should be a few cms. above the ground.

**What are the beneficial effects ?**

Basically, it is a relaxing posture. The abdomen is pressed against the ground, and therefore, with the movement of each deep breath, massage is given to the abdominal organs.

# KAPALBHATI

**What does the word Kapalbhati mean and what is this practice for?**

The synonym for this practice is 'diaphragmatic breathing' or 'bellow type breathing'. It is also called 'Sinus Cleanser'. The word 'Kapala' means forehead and 'Bhati' means to 'shine'. This practice involves rapid and forceful inhalations and exhalations and they help to clear the respiratory passages.

**I suppose when we breathe in this manner, it's like working the bellows?**

Yes, that is why it is called 'bellow-breathing'. Actually there is an up and down movement of the diaphragm which goes up while the belly is pushed in during exhalation and exactly the opposite during inhalation. Of course, the air is thrown in and out through the nose.

**How is this practised?**

You start with the Padmasana pose or any other similar pose.

**And then?**

Then placing the hands on the knee, you try to get into the breathing rhythm.

**How is that done?**

This is done by simply breathing in and out three or four times.

Next, (1) you raise the ribs and so expand the chest.

(2) You give an inward abdominal thrust—at the navel level,

(3) but you do so with a rapid and forceful exhalation through the nose with the mouth closed, and

(4) you will now relax the abdomen quickly, and simultaneously inhale through the nose.

**How often do you have to do that?**

About ten times, after which you lower the ribs and your one round is complete.

**Doesn't that mean you spend a lot of time on this practice?**

I wouldn't say that, because with practice the frequency in each round, as well as the number of rounds can be increased. Anyway, you remove the hands from the knees, and release the asana.

**What is your advice on what should or should not be done?**

A few precautions like (1) sitting erect and inhaling immediately after exhalation is over, and vice versa, (2) restricting the movement of the chest whilst breathing in and out, and (3) of course, keeping the mouth closed whilst breathing through the nose, are necessary.

**All these are 'shoulds', and what about the 'should nots'**

What I have said above includes the 'should nots' too, but there are a few 'don'ts' like:

1.  No 'thrust' to be given to the upper part of the abdomen.
2.  No contortions of the face are permitted.
3.  No backward or forward movements of the body during the respiratory action.
4.  No loading of the stomach with food prior to this practice and,
5.  Don't increase the speed of breathing unless you are able to establish good coordination between respiratory action and abdominal movements.

**What good is this practice to your body ?**

That it clears the respiratory passages is obvious, and therefore, for preventing lung infections, this is the best exercise. Again, the diaphragm is exercised enough and this promotes circulation.

*One last word:*

If you have acidity or ulcer trouble or for that matter any abdominal problem, you must take your doctor's O.K. before launching on this practice.

# ANULOMA VILOMA

**Do you have any special breathing exercise?**

Yes, but before I talk about this particular practice let me tell you that this is just one of the varieties of pranayama, i.e. breathing exercise. Actually there are three phases in a full pranayama. There is inhalation or breathing in. There is retention or holding the breath and there is exhalation or breathing out.

**In this variety which you call Anuloma Viloma which of these three aspects is most important?**

In Anuloma Viloma we lay emphasis on controlled inhalation and exhalation in the beginning and retention may be added later on. Now let's get on with the starting position, shall we?

**Yes, indeed.**

So, here we go.

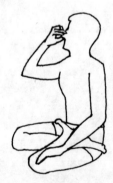

*Stage 1:* Sit comfortably in a pose like the Padmasana, or Swastikasana or in any suitable pose.
*Stage 2:* Sit erect with your hands on the knees.
*Stage 3:* Raising the right hand, close the index and middle fingers keeping the thumb and the last two fingers stretched out.
*Stage 4:* Closing the right nostril with the right thumb, inhale through the left nostril.

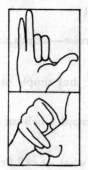 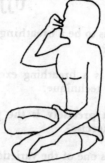

*Stage 5:* When the inhalation is over, you close the left nostril with the last two fingers and exhale through the right nostril, removing of course the right thumb.

*Stage 6:* After complete exhalation, inhale slowly through the same nostril — the right nostril.

*Stage 7:* Once again close the right nostril and exhale through the left nostril, removing of course, the last two fingers from the left nostril.

Thus repeat the last four stages, three to six, ten times or even more if you feel comfortable.

## What are the important points to remember here?

1. Inhalation must be gradual, allowing the air to be drawn in slowly.
2. Full exhalation is possible when you contract the abdominal muscles.

## But how long does one inhale and exhale?

Roughly 5 seconds for inhalation and 10 seconds for exhalation, maintaining this ratio of 1 to 2. Of course, you must *not* produce any sound from the nose.

Also don't press the nostril too much and avoid the temptation of holding the breath too long in the beginning.

I need not tell you that this exercise —
— brings you tranquillity and peace of mind,
— removes mental fatigue, and
— improves, of course, respiratory efficiency.

# UJJAYI

**This seems to be a breathing exercise—sounds simple too, doesn't it?**

Yes, it is a breathing exercise, but simple only if you follow the technique.

**But what precisely is the philosophy behind this particular exercise?**

Ujjayi is one of the varieties of what we call Pranayama. As you know, normally man goes on breathing, but when you voluntarily control this breathing, it becomes a pranayama.

**But why should there be any interference with nature's method of breathing?**

You will understand this when you examine carefully, the three actions that are involved, viz.—inhalation, holding the breath, and exhalation. Now, when you talk of holding the breath, it is obvious that you bring in voluntary control, but even while taking in fresh air and breathing out foul air you also bring in voluntary control.

**But don't you think that this voluntary control does affect, and perhaps even harm the normal breathing system?**

Well, in the beginning, during the phase of breath holding there is a possibility of undue strain on the delicate respiratory organs and mechanism leading to complications. That's why a beginner practises voluntary control on inhaling and exhaling only and in this particular pranayama, viz. Ujjayi, breath holding is avoided in the beginning.

**But what then is the speciality of this Ujjayi?**

The special characteristic of this pranayama is the frictional sound produced by contraction of the *glottis*.

**Glottis? What is this glottis?**

It is the sound producing apparatus of the larynx. Anyway, the special feature of the Ujjayi is that it can be practised in any comfortable position, sitting in any meditative posture (Padmasana, Swastikasana, Sukhasana etc.), and also while standing.

**But these are the famous meditative poses—Are't they?**

Yes, they are.

**What happens next?**

1. Placing your hands comfortably on your knees, you close the mouth and inhale slowly through both nostrils in a smooth uniform manner.
2. Keep the glottis partially closed and produce a frictional sound from the glottis.
3. Of course, this is done while breathing in, but take care not to allow the abdomen to bulge.
4. Now exhale slowly and contract the abdomen gradually, making the frictional sound from the glottis, and that completes one round of Ujjayi.

**How often is this done?**     About 7 to 10 times.

**What other precautions are to be taken?**

Some of the usual 'Dos' and 'Don'ts' I have already told you. However, (1) Try to maintain the time ratio of 1:2 between inhalation and exhalation, i.e. if you inhale for five seconds, take 10 seconds to exhale.

(2) The movement of the abdominal muscles must be under full control.

(3) A practical suggestion is that you close your eyes and concentrate on the flow of breath.

(4) Don't use your mouth either to inhale or exhale.

**And what happens after all this long winded routine?**

Ah! The practice of Ujjayi has a soothing effect on the body. It calms the mind, removes tensions and improves the respiratory efficiency.

## TABLE A

### PROXIMATE PRINCIPLES, MINERALS AND VITAMINS
### VALUES PER 100 GMS OF EDIBLE PORTION

Na = Sodium  
K = Potassium  
Mg = Magnesium

| S. No. | Name of foodstuff | Edible portion % | Moisture gm. | Protein gm. | Fat gm. | Fibre gm. | Carbo-hydrates gm. | Energy Kcal | Na mg | K mg | Mg mg | Cholesterol mg | Vitamin C mg |
|---|---|---|---|---|---|---|---|---|---|---|---|---|---|
| | | 1 | 2 | 3 | 4 | 5 | 6 | 7 | 8 | 9 | 10 | 11 | 12 |
| | **CEREAL GRAINS AND PRODUCTS** | | | | | | | | | | | | |
| 1. | Bajra (Pennisetum typhoideum) | 84 | 12 | 12 | 5 | 1 | 67 | 361 | 11 | 307 | 125 | | 0 |
| 2. | Barley (Hordeum vulgare) | 100 | 12 | 12 | 2 | | 70 | 336 | 16 | 253 | 127 | | 0 |
| 3. | Jowar (Sorghum vulgare) | 100 | 12 | 10 | 2 | | 73 | 349 | 7 | 131 | 140 | | 0 |
| 4. | Maize, dry (Zea mays) | 100 | 15 | 11 | 4 | | 66 | 342 | 16 | 286 | 144 | | 0 |
| 5. | Maize, tender (Zea mays) | 37 | 67 | 5 | 2 | | 25 | 125 | 52 | 151 | 40 | | 6 |
| 6. | Oatmeal (Avena byzantina) | 100 | 11 | 14 | 8 | 3 | 63 | 374 | | | | | 0 |
| 7. | Ragi (Eleusine coracana) | 100 | 13 | 7 | 1 | 4 | 72 | 328 | 11 | 408 | 191 | | 0 |
| 8. | Rice, pounded, handpounded (Oryza Sativa) | 100 | 13 | 8 | 1 | | 77 | 349 | | | | | 0 |
| 9. | Rice, parboiled, milled (Oryza Sativa) | 100 | 13 | 6 | 0 | 0 | 79 | 346 | 10 | 117 | 38 | | 0 |
| 10. | Rice, raw, handpounded | 100 | 13 | 7 | 1 | 1 | 77 | 346 | | | | | 0 |

PROXIMATE PRINCIPLES, MINERALS AND VITAMINS
VALUES PER 100 GMS OF EDIBLE PORTION

K = Potassium
Mg = Magnesium

| S. No. | Name of foodstuff | Edible portion % | Moisture gm. | Protein gm. | Fat gm. | Fibre gm. | Carbo-hydrates gm. | Energy Kcal | Na mg | K mg | Mg mg | Cholesterol mg | Vitamin C mg |
|---|---|---|---|---|---|---|---|---|---|---|---|---|---|
| | | 1 | 2 | 3 | 4 | 5 | 6 | 7 | 8 | 9 | 10 | 11 | 12 |
| 11. | Rice, raw, milled (Oryza Sativa) | 100 | 14 | 7 | 0 | 0 | 78 | 345 | 8 | 70 | 48 | | 0 |
| 12. | Rice bran (Oryza Sativa) | .. | 11 | 13 | 16 | 4 | 48 | 393 | | | | | 0 |
| 13. | Rice flakes (Oryza Sativa) | 100 | 12 | 7 | 1 | 1 | 77 | 346 | 11 | 154 | 101 | | 0 |
| 14. | Rice, puffed (Oryza Sativa) | 100 | 15 | 7 | 0 | 0 | 74 | 325 | | | | | 0 |
| 15. | Vermicelli (Triticum aestivum) | 100 | 12 | 9 | | — | 78 | 352 | 8 | 138 | 42 | | 0 |
| 16. | Wheat (whole) (Triticum aestivum) | 100 | 13 | 12 | 1 | 1 | 71 | 346 | 17 | 284 | 138 | | 0 |
| 17. | Wheat flour (whole) (Triticum aestivum) | 100 | 12 | 12 | 2 | 2 | 69 | 341 | 20 | 315 | 55 | | 0 |
| 18. | Wheat flour (refined) (Triticum aestivum) | 100 | 13 | 11 | 1 | 0 | 74 | 348 | 9 | 130 | 42 | | 0 |
| 19. | Wheat germ (Triticum aestivum) | 100 | 5 | 29 | 7 | 1 | 53 | 397 | | | | | 0 |

## TABLE B

### PROXIMATE PRINCIPLES, MINERALS AND VITAMINS VALUES PER 100 GMS OF EDIBLE PORTION

Na = Sodium
K = Potassium
Mg = Magnesium

| S. No. | Name of foodstuff | Edible portion % | Moisture gm. | Protein gm. | Fat gm. | Fibre gm. | Carbo-hydrates gm. | Energy Kcal | Na mg | K mg | Mg mg | Cholesterol mg | Vitamin C mg |
|---|---|---|---|---|---|---|---|---|---|---|---|---|---|
| | | 1 | 2 | 3 | 4 | 5 | 6 | 7 | 8 | 9 | 10 | 11 | 12 |
| **PULSES AND LEGUMES** | | | | | | | | | | | | | |
| 20. | Bengal gram (whole) Cicer arietinum | 100 | 10 | 17 | 5 | 4 | 61 | 360 | 37 | 808 | 168 | | 3 |
| 21. | Bengal gram dhal Cicer arietinum | 100 | 10 | 21 | 6 | 1 | 60 | 372 | 73 | 720 | 138 | | 1 |
| 22. | Bengal gram (Roasted) Cicer arietinum | 100 | 11 | 22 | 5 | 1 | 58 | 369 | | | | | 0 |
| 23. | Black gram dhal Phaseolus mungo | 100 | 11 | 24 | 1 | 1 | 60 | 347 | 40 | 800 | 185 | | 0 |
| 24. | Green gram (whole) Phaseolus aureus Roxb | 100 | 10 | 24 | 1 | 4 | 57 | 334 | 28 | 843 | 171 | | 0 |
| 25. | Green gram dhal Phaseolus aureus Roxb | 100 | 10 | 24 | 1 | 1 | 60 | 348 | 27 | 1150 | 189 | | 0 |
| 26. | Lentil Lens esculenta | 100 | 12 | 25 | 1 | 1 | 59 | 343 | 40 | 629 | 94 | | 0 |
| 27. | Peas, dry Pisum sativum | 100 | 16 | 20 | 1 | 4 | 56 | 315 | 20 | 725 | 124 | | 0 |
| 28. | Peas, roasted | 100 | | | | | | | | | | | |

## TABLE B
### PROXIMATE PRINCIPLES, MINERALS AND VITAMINS VALUES PER 100 GMS OF EDIBLE PORTION

| S. No. | Name of foodstuff | Edible portion % | Moisture gm. | Protein gm. | Fat gm. | Fibre gm. | Carbo-hydrates gm. | Energy Kcal | Na mg | K mg | Mg mg | Cholesterol mg | Vitamin C mg |
|---|---|---|---|---|---|---|---|---|---|---|---|---|---|
|  |  | 1 | 2 | 3 | 4 | 5 | 6 | 7 | 8 | 9 | 10 | 11 | 12 |
| 29. | Rajmah (Phaseolus vulgaris) | — | 12 | 23 | 1 | — | 61 | 346 |  |  |  |  | — |
| 30. | Redgram dhal (Cajanus cajan) | 100 | 13 | 22 | 2 | 1 | 58 | 335 | 28 | 1104 | 133 |  | 0 |
| 31. | Soyabean (Glycine max Merr) | — | 8 | 43 | 19 | 4 | 21 | 432 |  |  |  |  | — |

## TABLE C
### PROXIMATE PRINCIPLES, MINERALS AND VITAMINS VALUES PER 100 GMS OF EDIBLE PORTION

Na = Sodium
K = Potassium
Mg = Magnesium

| S. No. | Name of foodstuff | Edible portion % | Moisture gm. | Protein gm. | Fat gm. | Fibre gm. | Carbo-hydrates gm. | Energy Kcal | Na mg | K mg | Mg mg | Cholesterol mg | Vitamin C mg |
|---|---|---|---|---|---|---|---|---|---|---|---|---|---|
| | | 1 | 2 | 3 | 4 | 5 | 6 | 7 | 8 | 9 | 10 | 11 | 12 |
| **LEAFY VEGETABLES** | | | | | | | | | | | | | |
| 32. | Amaranth, spined (Amaranthus spinosus) | — | 85 | 3 | 0 | 1 | 7 | 43 | | | | | 33 |
| 33. | Amaranth, tender (Amaranthus gangeticus) | 39 | 86 | 4 | 0 | 1 | 6 | 45 | 230 | 341 | 247 | | 99 |
| 34. | Ambat chuka (Rumex vesicarius) | — | 95 | 2 | 0 | 1 | 1 | 15 | | | | | 12 |
| 35. | Bamboo, tender shoots (Bambusa arundinacea) | 54 | 89 | 4 | 0 | — | 6 | 43 | 91 | — | 32 | | 5 |
| 36. | Bottle gourd leaves (Langenaria valgaris) | — | 88 | 2 | 1 | 1 | 6 | 39 | | | | | — |
| 37. | Broad bean leaves (Vicia faba) | — | 78 | 6 | 0 | 4 | 11 | 71 | | | | | — |
| 38. | Brussels sprouts (Brassica oleracea var gemmifera) | 100 | 85 | 5 | 0 | 1 | 7 | 52 | 8 | 477 | 26 | | 72 |
| 39. | Cabbage (Brassica oleracea var capitata) | 88 | 92 | 2 | 0 | 1 | 5 | 27 | 14 | 114 | 10 | | 124 |
| 40. | Carrot leaves (Daucus carota) | 51 | 77 | 5 | 0 | 2 | 13 | 77 | | | | | 79 |

TABLE C

PROXIMATE PRINCIPLES, MINERALS AND VITAMINS
VALUES PER 100 GMS OF EDIBLE PORTION

Na = Sodium
K = Potassium
Mg = Magnesium

| S. No. | Name of foodstuff | Edible portion % | Moisture gm. | Protein gm. | Fat gm. | Fibre gm. | Carbo-hydrates gm. | Energy Kcal | Na mg | K mg | Mg mg | Cholesterol mg | Vitamin C mg |
|---|---|---|---|---|---|---|---|---|---|---|---|---|---|
| | | 1 | 2 | 3 | 4 | 5 | 6 | 7 | 8 | 9 | 10 | 11 | 12 |
| 41. | Cauliflower greens (Brassica Oleracea var botrytis) | — | 80 | 6 | 1 | 2 | 8 | 66 | 4 | 18 | 8 | | — |
| 42. | Celery leaves (Apium graveolens var dulce) | 71 | 88 | 6 | 1 | 1 | 2 | 37 | 35 | 210 | 52 | | 62 |
| 43. | Colocasia leaves (black-variety) (Colocasia antiquorum) | — | 79 | 7 | 2 | 2 | 8 | 77 | | | | | 63 |
| 44. | Coriander leaves (Coriandrum sativum) | 70 | 86 | 3 | 1 | 1 | 6 | 44 | 58 | 256 | 64 | | 135 |
| 45. | Curry leaves (Murraya Koenigii) | 83 | 64 | 6 | 1 | 6 | 19 | 108 | — | — | 221 | | 4 |
| 46. | Drumstick leaves (Moringa oleifera) | 75 | 76 | 7 | 2 | 1 | 12 | 92 | — | 259 | 24 | | 220 |
| 47. | Fenugreek leaves (Trigonella foenumgraecum) | 59 | 86 | 4 | 1 | 1 | 6 | 49 | 76 | 31 | 67 | | 52 |
| 48. | Knol-khol greens (Brassica oleracea var caulorapa) | 73 | 87 | 3 | 0 | 2 | 6 | 43 | | | | | 157 |
| 49. | Lettuce (Lactuca sativa) | 66 | 93 | 2 | 0 | 0 | 2 | 21 | 58 | 33 | 30 | | 10 |
| 50. | Lettuce tree leaves, mature (Pisonia alba) | — | 82 | 5 | 0 | — | 10 | 65 | | | | | — |

TABLE C

PROXIMATE PRINCIPLES, MINERALS AND VITAMINS
VALUES PER 100 GMS OF EDIBLE PORTION

| S. No. | Name of foodstuff | Edible portion % | Moisture gm. | Protein gm. | Fat gm. | Fibre gm. | Carbo-hydrates gm. | Energy Kcal | Na mg | K mg | Mg mg | Cholesterol mg | Vitamin C mg |
|---|---|---|---|---|---|---|---|---|---|---|---|---|---|
| | | 1 | 2 | 3 | 4 | 5 | 6 | 7 | 8 | 9 | 10 | 11 | 12 |
| 51. | Lettuce tree leaves, tender (Pisonia alba) | — | 90 | 4 | 0 | 1 | 3 | 29 | 9 | 240 | 8 | | 10 |
| 52. | Mint (Mentha spicata) | 45 | 85 | 5 | 1 | 2 | 6 | 48 | — | — | — | | 27 |
| 53. | Parsley (Petroselinum crispum) | 82 | 75 | 6 | 1 | 2 | 13 | 87 | 33 | 1080 | 52 | | 281 |
| 54. | Parwar sag (Trichosanthes dioica) | — | 80 | 5 | 1 | 4 | 6 | 55 | | | | | — |
| 55. | Potato leaves (Solanum tuberosum) | — | 88 | 4 | 1 | 1 | 4 | 40 | | | | | — |
| 56. | Pumpkin leaves (Cucurbita maxima) | — | 82 | 5 | 1 | 2 | 8 | 57 | | | | | — |
| 57. | Radish leaves (Raphanus sativus) | 100 | 91 | 4 | 0 | 1 | 2 | 28 | | | | | 81 |
| 58. | Safflower leaves (Carthamus tinctorius) | 66 | 91 | 2 | 1 | — | 4 | 33 | 126 | 181 | 51 | | 15 |
| 59. | Spinach (Spinacia oleracea) | 87 | 92 | 2 | 1 | 1 | 3 | 26 | 58 | 206 | 84 | | 28 |
| 60. | Sweet potato greens | 100 | 81 | 4 | 1 | 2 | 10 | 61 | | | | | |

TABLE C

PROXIMATE PRINCIPLES, MINERALS AND VITAMINS
VALUES PER 100 GMS OF EDIBLE PORTION

| S. No. | Name of foodstuff | Edible portion % | Moisture gm. | Protein gm. | Fat gm. | Fibre gm. | Carbo-hydrates gm. | Energy Kcal | Na mg | K mg | Mg mg | Cholesterol mg | Vitamin C mg |
|---|---|---|---|---|---|---|---|---|---|---|---|---|---|
| | | 1 | 2 | 3 | 4 | 5 | 6 | 7 | 8 | 9 | 10 | 11 | 12 |
| 61. | Table radish leaves (Raphanus sativus) | 49 | 89 | 4 | 1 | 1 | 4 | 38 | | | | | 106 |
| 62. | Tamarind leaves, tender, dried (Tamarindus indicus) | — | 9 | 9 | 3 | 10 | 61 | 305 | — | — | 71 | | — |
| 63. | Turnip greens (Brassica rapa) | 51 | 82 | 4 | 1 | 1 | 9 | 67 | | | | | 180 |

## TABLE D
### PROXIMATE PRINCIPLES, MINERALS AND VITAMINS
### VALUES PER 100 GMS OF EDIBLE PORTION

Na = Sodium
K = Potassium
Mg = Magnesium

| S. No. | Name of foodstuff | Edible portion % | Moisture gm. | Protein gm. | Fat gm. | Fibre gm. | Carbo-hydrates gm. | Energy Kcal | Na mg | K mg | Mg mg | Cholesterol mg | Vitamin C mg |
|---|---|---|---|---|---|---|---|---|---|---|---|---|---|
| | | 1 | 2 | 3 | 4 | 5 | 6 | 7 | 8 | 9 | 10 | 11 | 12 |
| ROOTS AND TUBERS | | | | | | | | | | | | | |
| 64. | Beet root (Beta vulgaris) | 85 | 88 | 2 | 0 | 1 | 9 | 43 | 60 | 43 | 9 | — | 10 |
| 65. | Carrot (Daucus carota) | 95 | 86 | 1 | 0 | 1 | 11 | 48 | 36 | 108 | 14 | | 3 |
| 66. | Onion big (Allium cepa) | 95 | 87 | 1 | 0 | 1 | 11 | 50 | | | | | 11 |
| 67. | Onion, small (Allium cepa) | — | 84 | 2 | 0 | 1 | 13 | 59 | 4 | 127 | — | | 2 |
| 68. | Potato (Solanum tuberosum) | 85 | 75 | 2 | 0 | 0 | 23 | 97 | 11 | 247 | 20 | | 17 |
| 69. | Radish, pink (Raphanus sativus) | 98 | 91 | 1 | 0 | 1 | 7 | 32 | 63 | 10 | 9 | | 17 |
| 70. | Radish table (Raphanus sativus) | 100 | 95 | 0 | 0 | 1 | 3 | 16 | | | | | 21 |
| 71. | Radish, white (Raphanus sativus) | 99 | 94 | 1 | 0 | 1 | 3 | 17 | 33 | 138 | | | 15 |
| 72. | Sweet potato (Ipomoea batatas) | 97 | 68 | 1 | 0 | 1 | 28 | 120 | 9 | 393 | | | 24 |
| 73. | Tapioca (Manihot esculenta) | — | 59 | 1 | 0 | 1 | 38 | 157 | | | | | 25 |

## TABLE D
### PROXIMATE PRINCIPLES, MINERALS AND VITAMINS
### VALUES PER 100 GMS OF EDIBLE PORTION

Na = Sodium
K = Potassium
Mg = Magnesium

| S. No. | Name of foodstuff | Edible portion % | Moisture gm. | Protein gm. | Fat gm. | Fibre gm. | Carbo-hydrates gm. | Energy Kcal | Na mg | K mg | Mg mg | Cholesterol mg | Vitamin C mg |
|---|---|---|---|---|---|---|---|---|---|---|---|---|---|
| | | 1 | 2 | 3 | 4 | 5 | 6 | 7 | 8 | 9 | 10 | 11 | 12 |
| 74. | Turnip (Brassica rapa) | 65 | 92 | 0 | 0 | 1 | 6 | 29 | | | | | 43 |
| 75. | Yam, wild (Dioscorea versicolor) | 89 | 70 | 2 | 0 | 1 | 24 | 110 | 11 | 450 | 34 | | 1 |

## TABLE E
### PROXIMATE PRINCIPLES, MINERALS AND VITAMINS
#### VALUES PER 100 GMS OF EDIBLE PORTION

Na = Sodium
K = Potassium
Mg = Magnesium

| S. No. | Name of foodstuff | Edible portion % | Moisture gm. | Protein gm. | Fat gm. | Fibre gm. | Carbo-hydrates gm. | Energy Kcal | Na mg | K mg | Mg mg | Cholesterol mg | Vitamin C mg |
|---|---|---|---|---|---|---|---|---|---|---|---|---|---|
| | | 1 | 2 | 3 | 4 | 5 | 6 | 7 | 8 | 9 | 10 | 11 | 12 |
| OTHER VEGETABLES | | | | | | | | | | | | | |
| 76. | Artichoke (Cynara Scolymus) | — | 77 | 4 | 0 | 1 | 16 | 79 | | | | | 0 |
| 77. | Bitter gourd (Momordica Charantia) | 97 | 92 | 2 | 0 | 1 | 4 | 25 | 18 | 152 | 17 | | 88 |
| 78. | Brinjal (Solanum melongena) | 91 | 93 | 1 | 0 | 1 | 4 | 24 | 3 | 200 | 16 | | 12 |
| 79. | Broad beans (Vicia faba) | 88 | 85 | 4 | 0 | 2 | 7 | 48 | 43 | 39 | 33 | | 12 |
| 80. | Cauliflower (Brassica oleracea var) | 70 | 91 | 3 | 0 | 1 | 4 | 30 | 53 | 138 | 20 | | 56 |
| 81. | Celery stalks (Apium graveolens var. dulce) | — | 93 | 1 | 0 | 1 | 3 | 18 | | | | | 6 |
| 82. | Cluster beans (Cyamopsis tetragonoloba) | — | 81 | 3 | 0 | 3 | 11 | 60 | | | | | 49 |
| 83. | Cucumber (Cucumis sativus) | 83 | 96 | 0 | 0 | 0 | 2 | 13 | 10 | 50 | 11 | | 7 |
| 84. | Double beans | — | 74 | 8 | 0 | 4 | 12 | 85 | | | | | 32 |

TABLE E

PROXIMATE PRINCIPLES, MINERALS AND VITAMINS
VALUES PER 100 GMS OF EDIBLE PORTION

K = Potassium
Mg = Magnesium

| S.No. | Name of foodstuff | Edible portion % | Moisture gm. | Protein gm. | Fat gm. | Fibre gm. | Carbohydrates gm. | Energy Kcal | Na mg | K mg | Mg mg | Cholesterol mg | Vitamin C mg |
|---|---|---|---|---|---|---|---|---|---|---|---|---|---|
| | | 1 | 2 | 3 | 4 | 5 | 6 | 7 | 8 | 9 | 10 | 11 | 12 |
| OTHER VEGETABLES | | | | | | | | | | | | | |
| 85. | Drumstick (Moringa oleifera) | 83 | 87 | 2 | 0 | 5 | 4 | 26 | — | 259 | 24 | | 120 |
| 86. | French beans (Phaseolus vulgaris) | 94 | 91 | 2 | 0 | 2 | 4 | 26 | 4 | 120 | 29 | | 24 |
| 87. | Giant Chillies (capsicum) (Capsicum annuum var. grossa) | 97 | 92 | 1 | 0 | 1 | 4 | 24 | | | | | 137 |
| 88. | Knol-khol (Brassica oleracea var. caulorapa) | 74 | 93 | 2 | 0 | 1 | 4 | 21 | 112 | 37 | 18 | | 85 |
| 89. | Ladies fingers (Abelmoschus esculentus) | 84 | 90 | 2 | 0 | 1 | 6 | 35 | 7 | 103 | 43 | | 13 |
| 90. | Leeks (Allium porrum) | — | 79 | 2 | 0 | 1 | 17 | 77 | | | | | 11 |
| 91. | Mango, green (Mangsfera indica) | 72 | 87 | 1 | 0 | 1 | 10 | 44 | 43 | 83 | 21 | | 3 |
| 92. | Onion stalks (Allium cepa) | 100 | 88 | 1 | 0 | 2 | 9 | 41 | 2 | 109 | 15 | | 17 |
| 93. | Papaya, green (Carica papaya) | — | 92 | 1 | 0 | 1 | 6 | 27 | 23 | 216 | — | | 12 |

# TABLE E
## PROXIMATE PRINCIPLES, MINERALS AND VITAMINS
### VALUES PER 100 GMS OF EDIBLE PORTION

Na = Sodium
K = Potassium
Mg = Magnesium

| S. No. | Name of foodstuff | Edible portion % | Moisture gm. | Protein gm. | Fat gm. | Fibre gm. | Carbo-hydrates gm. | Energy Kcal | Na mg | K mg | Mg mg | Cholesterol mg | Vitamin C mg |
|---|---|---|---|---|---|---|---|---|---|---|---|---|---|
| | | 1 | 2 | 3 | 4 | 5 | 6 | 7 | 8 | 9 | 10 | 11 | 12 |
| OTHER VEGETABLES | | | | | | | | | | | | | |
| 94. | Parwar (Trichosanthes dioica) | 95 | 92 | 2 | 0 | 3 | 2 | 20 | 3 | 83 | 9 | | 29 |
| 95. | Peas (Pisum sativum) | 53 | 72 | 7 | 0 | 4 | 16 | 93 | 8 | 79 | 34 | | 9 |
| 96. | Plantain, green (Musa sapientum) | 58 | 83 | 1 | 0 | 1 | 14 | 64 | 15 | 193 | 33 | | 24 |
| 97. | Pumpkin (Cucurbita maxima) | 79 | 93 | 1 | 0 | 1 | 5 | 25 | 6 | 139 | 14 | | 2 |
| 98. | Rhubarb stalks (Rheum emodi) | — | 93 | | 0 | 0 | 4 | 26 | | | | | 37 |
| 99. | Ridge gourd (Luffa acutangula) | 82 | 95 | 0 | 0 | 0 | 3 | 17 | 3 | 50 | 11 | | 5 |
| 100. | Snake gourd (Tricosanthes anguina) | 98 | 95 | 0 | 0 | 1 | 3 | 18 | 25 | 34 | 53 | | 0 |
| 101. | Spinach stalks (Spinacia oleracea) | — | 93 | 0 | 0 | — | 4 | 20 | | | | | 3 |
| 102. | Tinda, tender (Citrullus vulgaris var fistulosus) | 99 | 93 | 1 | 0 | 1 | 3 | 21 | 35 | 24 | 14 | | 18 |
| 103. | Tomato, green (Lycopersicon esculentum) | 98 | 93 | 2 | 0 | 1 | 4 | 23 | 46 | 114 | 15 | | 31 |

PROXIMATE PRINCIPLES, MINERALS AND VITAMINS
VALUES PER 100 GMS OF EDIBLE PORTION

K = Potassium
Mg = Magnesium

| S. No. | Name of foodstuff | Edible portion % | Moisture gm. | Protein gm. | Fat gm. | Fibre gm. | Carbo-hydrates gm. | Energy Kcal | Na mg | K mg | Mg mg | Cholesterol mg | Vitamin C mg |
|---|---|---|---|---|---|---|---|---|---|---|---|---|---|
| | | 1 | 2 | 3 | 4 | 5 | 6 | 7 | 8 | 9 | 10 | 11 | 12 |
| NUTS AND SEEDS | | | | | | | | | | | | | |
| 104. | Almond (Prunus amygdalus) | — | 5 | 21 | 59 | 2 | 10 | 655 | 6 | 250 | 260 | | 0 |
| 105. | Cashewnut (Anacardium occidentale) | — | 6 | 21 | 47 | 1 | 22 | 596 | | | | | 0 |
| 106. | Chilgoza (Pinus gerardiana) | — | 4 | 14 | 49 | 1 | 29 | 615 | | | | | 0 |
| 107. | Coconut, dry (Cocos nucifera) | — | 4 | 7 | 62 | 7 | 18 | 662 | | | | | 7 |
| 108. | Coconut, fresh (Cocos nucifera) | 100 | 36 | 4 | 42 | 4 | 13 | 444 | | | | | 1 |
| 109. | Gingelly seeds (Sesamum indicum) | 100 | 5 | 18 | 43 | 3 | 25 | 563 | | | | | 0 |
| 110. | Groundnut (Arachis hypogaea) | 73 | 3 | 25 | 40 | 3 | 26 | 567 | | | | | 0 |
| 111. | Groundnut, roasted (Arachis hypogaea) | 69 | 2 | 26 | 40 | 3 | 27 | 570 | | | | | 0 |
| 112. | Mustard seeds (Brassica nigra) | — | 8 | 20 | 40 | 2 | 24 | 541 | | | | | 0 |

## TABLE F
### PROXIMATE PRINCIPLES, MINERALS AND VITAMINS VALUES PER 100 GMS OF EDIBLE PORTION

Na = Sodium
K = Potassium
Mg = Magnesium

| S. No. | Name of foodstuff | Edible portion % | Moisture gm. | Protein gm. | Fat gm. | Fibre gm. | Carbo-hydrates gm. | Energy Kcal | Na mg | K mg | Mg mg | Cholesterol mg | Vitamin C mg |
|---|---|---|---|---|---|---|---|---|---|---|---|---|---|
| | | 1 | 2 | 3 | 4 | 5 | 6 | 7 | 8 | 9 | 10 | 11 | 12 |
| **NUTS AND SEEDS** | | | | | | | | | | | | | |
| 113. | Pistachio nut (Pistacia vera) | — | 6 | 20 | 53 | 2 | 16 | 626 | | | | | 12 |
| 114. | Safflower seeds (Carthamus tinctorius) | — | 5 | 13 | 26 | 35 | 18 | 356 | | | | | — |
| 115. | Sunflower seeds (Halianthus annuus) | 52 | 5 | 20 | 52 | 1 | 18 | 620 | | | | | 1 |
| 116. | Walnut (Juglans regia) | 45 | 4 | 16 | 64 | 3 | 11 | 687 | 3 | 690 | 130 | | 0 |

PROXIMATE PRINCIPLES, MINERALS AND VITAMINS
VALUES PER 100 GMS OF EDIBLE PORTION

K = Potassium
Mg = Magnesium

| S. No. | Name of foodstuff | Edible portion % | Moisture gm. | Protein gm. | Fat gm. | Fibre gm. | Carbo-hydrates gm. | Energy Kcal | Na mg | K mg | Mg mg | Cholesterol mg | Vitamin C mg |
|---|---|---|---|---|---|---|---|---|---|---|---|---|---|
| | | 1 | 2 | 3 | 4 | 5 | 6 | 7 | 8 | 9 | 10 | 11 | 12 |
| CONDIMENTS, SPICES ETC. | | | | | | | | | | | | | |
| 117. | Asafoetida (Ferula foetida) | — | 16 | 4 | 1 | 4 | 68 | 297 | | | | | 0 |
| 118. | Cardamom (Elettaria cardamomum) | — | 20 | 10 | 2 | 20 | 42 | 229 | | | | | 0 |
| 119. | Chillies, dry (Capsicum annuum) | — | 10 | 16 | 6 | 30 | 32 | 246 | 14 | 530 | — | | 50 |
| 120. | Chillies, green (Capsicum annuum) | 90 | 86 | 3 | 1 | 7 | 3 | 29 | 6 | 217 | 24 | | 111 |
| 121. | Cloves, dry (Syzygium aromaticum) | 100 | 25 | 5 | 9 | 9 | 46 | 286 | | | | | 0 |
| 122. | Cloves, green (Syzygium aromaticum) | — | 65 | 2 | 6 | — | 24 | 159 | | | | | — |
| 123. | Coriander (Coriandrum sativum) | — | 11 | 14 | 16 | 33 | 22 | 288 | 32 | 990 | — | | 0 |
| 124. | Cumin seeds (Cuminum cyminum) | — | 12 | 19 | 15 | 12 | 37 | 356 | 126 | 980 | — | | 3 |
| 125. | Fenugreek seeds (Trigonella foenum-graecum) | — | 14 | 26 | 6 | 7 | 44 | 333 | 19 | 530 | — | | 0 |
| 126. | Garlic, dry (Allium sativum) | 85 | 62 | 6 | 0 | 1 | 30 | 145 | | | | | 13 |

TABLE G

## PROXIMATE PRINCIPLES, MINERALS AND VITAMINS VALUES PER 100 GMS OF EDIBLE PORTION

Na = Sodium
K = Potassium
Mg = Magnesium

| S. No. | Name of foodstuff | Edible portion % | Moisture gm. | Protein gm. | Fat gm. | Fibre gm. | Carbo-hydrates gm. | Energy Kcal | Na mg | K mg | Mg. mg | Cholesterol mg | Vitamin C mg |
|---|---|---|---|---|---|---|---|---|---|---|---|---|---|
| | | 1 | 2 | 3 | 4 | 5 | 6 | 7 | 8 | 9 | 10 | 11 | 12 |
| 127. | Ginger, fresh (Zingiber officinale) | — | 81 | 2 | 1 | 2 | 12 | 67 | | | | | 6 |
| 128. | Nutmeg (Myristica fragrans) | — | 14 | 7 | 36 | 12 | 28 | 472 | | | | | 0 |
| 129. | Pepper, dry (Piper nigrum) | 95 | 13 | 11 | 7 | 15 | 49 | 304 | | | | | — |
| 130. | Pepper, green (Piper nigrum) | 81 | 71 | 5 | 3 | 6 | 14 | 98 | | | | | 1 |
| 131. | Tamarind pulp (Tamarindus indica) | — | 21 | 3 | 0 | 6 | 67 | 283 | | | | | 3 |
| 132. | Turmeric (Curcuma domestica) | 100 | 13 | 6 | 5 | 3 | 69 | 349 | 25 | 3300 | — | | 0 |

PROXIMATE PRINCIPLES, MINERALS AND VITAMINS
VALUES PER 100 GMS OF EDIBLE PORTION

K = Potassium
Mg = Magnesium

| S. No. | Name of foodstuff | Edible portion % | Moisture gm. | Protein gm. | Fat gm. | Fibre gm. | Carbo-hydrates gm. | Energy Kcal | Na mg | K mg | Mg mg | Cholesterol mg | Vitamin C mg |
|---|---|---|---|---|---|---|---|---|---|---|---|---|---|
| | | 1 | 2 | 3 | 4 | 5 | 6 | 7 | 8 | 9 | 10 | 11 | 12 |
| **FRUITS** | | | | | | | | | | | | | |
| 133. | Amla (Emblica officinalis) | 89 | 82 | 0 | 0 | 3 | 14 | 58 | 5 | 225 | — | | 600 |
| 134. | Apple (Malus sylvestris) | 90 | 85 | 0 | 0 | 1 | 13 | 59 | 28 | 75 | 7 | | 1 |
| 135. | Apricots, fresh (Prunus armeniaca) | 86 | 85 | 1 | 0 | .1 | 12 | 53 | 56 | 430 | 65 | | 6 |
| 136. | Apricots, dried (Prunus armeniaca) | 93 | 19 | 2 | 1 | 2 | 73 | 306 | 2 | | | | 2 |
| 137. | Avocado pear (Persea americana) | — | 74 | 2 | 23 | — | 1 | 215 | 2 | 400 | 29 | | — |
| 138. | Bael fruit (Aegle Marmalos) | 64 | 61 | 2 | 0 | 3 | 32 | 137 | | | | | 8 |
| 139. | Bamboo fruit (Bambusa arundinacea) | — | 56 | 4 | 0 | 4 | 34 | 153 | | | | | 1 |
| 140. | Banana, ripe (Musa paradisiaca) | 71 | 70 | 1 | 0 | 0 | 27 | 116 | 37 | 88 | 34 | | 7 |
| 141. | Blackberry (Rubus fruiticosus) | 100 | 87 | 1 | 0 | 4 | 7 | 37 | | | | | 9 |
| 142. | Bread fruit (Artocarpus altilis) | — | 79 | 1 | 0 | 2 | 16 | 71 | | | | | 21 |

## TABLE H
### PROXIMATE PRINCIPLES, MINERALS AND VITAMINS
### VALUES PER 100 GMS OF EDIBLE PORTION

Na = Sodium
K = Potassium
Mg = Magnesium

| S. No. | Name of foodstuff | Edible portion % | Moisture gm. | Protein gm. | Fat gm. | Fibre gm. | Carbo-hydrates gm. | Energy Kcal | Na mg | K mg | Mg mg | Cholesterol mg | Vitamin C mg |
|---|---|---|---|---|---|---|---|---|---|---|---|---|---|
| | | 1 | 2 | 3 | 4 | 5 | 6 | 7 | 8 | 9 | 10 | 11 | 12 |
| 143. | Cashew fruit (Anacardium occidentale) | 77 | 86 | 0 | 0 | 1 | 12 | 51 | | | | | 180 |
| 144. | Cherries, red (Prunus cerasus) | 88 | 83 | 1 | 0 | 0 | 14 | 64 | 3 | 320 | 10 | | 7 |
| 145. | Cherimoyer (Annona cherimolia) | 73 | 76 | 1 | 0 | 1 | 20 | 89 | | | | | 7 |
| 146. | Currants, black | 98 | 18 | 3 | 0 | 1 | 75 | 316 | | | | | 1 |
| 147. | Dates, dried (Phoenix dactylifera) | 86 | 15 | 2 | 0 | 4 | 76 | 317 | 5 | 750 | 59 | | 3 |
| 148. | Dates, fresh (Phoenix dactylifera) | — | 59 | 1 | 0 | 4 | 34 | 144 | | | | | — |
| 149. | Figs (Ficus carica) | 99 | 88 | 1 | 0 | 2 | 8 | 37 | 2 | 270 | 20 | | 5 |
| 150. | Grapes, blue variety (Vitis vinifera) | 95 | 82 | 1 | 0 | 3 | 13 | 58 | | | | | 1 |
| 151. | Grapes, pale green variety (Vitis vinifera) | — | 79 | 0 | 0 | 3 | 16 | 71 | | | | | 1 |
| 152. | Grapefruit (Marsh's seedless) (Citrus paradisi) | — | 88 | 1 | 0 | — | 10 | 45 | | | | | — |
| 153. | Guava, country (Psidium guajava) | 100 | 82 | 1 | 0 | 5 | 11 | 51 | 5 | 91 | 8 | | 212 |

Na = Sodium
K = Potassium
Mg = Magnesium

## TABLE H

### PROXIMATE PRINCIPLES, MINERALS AND VITAMINS
### VALUES PER 100 GMS OF EDIBLE PORTION

| S. No. | Name of foodstuff | Edible portion % | Moisture gm. | Protein gm. | Fat gm. | Fibre gm. | Carbo-hydrates gm. | Energy Kcal | Na mg | K mg | Mg mg | Cholesterol mg | Vitamin C mg |
|---|---|---|---|---|---|---|---|---|---|---|---|---|---|
| | | 1 | 2 | 3 | 4 | 5 | 6 | 7 | 8 | 9 | 10 | 11 | 12 |
| 154. | Jack fruit (Artocarpus heterophyllus) | 30 | 76 | 2 | 0 | 1 | 20 | 88 | 41 | 191 | 27 | | 7 |
| 155. | Jambu fruit (Syzygium cumini) | 75 | 84 | 1 | 0 | 1 | 14 | 62 | 26 | 55 | 35 | | 18 |
| 156. | Lemon (Citrus limon) | — | 85 | 1 | 1 | 2 | 11 | 57 | — | 270 | — | | 39 |
| 157. | Lemon, sweet (Citrus limetta) | 79 | 90 | 1 | 0 | 1 | 7 | 35 | — | 210 | — | | 45 |
| 158. | Lichi (Nephelium litchi) | 68 | 84 | 1 | 0 | 0 | 14 | 61 | 125 | 159 | 10 | | 31 |
| 159. | Lichies, bastard (Nephelium longana) | — | 84 | 1 | 0 | 0 | 13 | 61 | | | | | — |
| 160. | Lime (Citrus aurantifolia) | — | 49 | 1 | 1 | 1 | 11 | 59 | | | | | 63 |
| 161. | Lime, sweet, musambi (Citrus sinensis) | 71 | 88 | 1 | 0 | 0 | 9 | 43 | — | 490 | — | | 50 |
| 162. | Mango, ripe (Mangifera indica) | 74 | 81 | 1 | 0 | 1 | 17 | 74 | 26 | 205 | 27 | | 16 |
| 163. | Melon, water (Citrullus vulgaris) | 78 | 96 | 0 | 0 | 0 | 3 | 16 | 27 | 160 | 13 | | 1 |

TABLE H

PROXIMATE PRINCIPLES, MINERALS AND VITAMINS
VALUES PER 100 GMS OF EDIBLE PORTION

| S. No. | Name of foodstuff | Edible portion % | Moisture gm. | Protein gm. | Fat gm. | Fibre gm. | Carbo-hydrates gm. | Energy Kcal | Na mg | K mg | Mg mg | Cholesterol mg | Vitamin C mg |
|---|---|---|---|---|---|---|---|---|---|---|---|---|---|
| | | 1 | 2 | 3 | 4 | 5 | 6 | 7 | 8 | 9 | 10 | 11 | 12 |
| 164. | Orange (Citrus aurantium) | 67 | 88 | 1 | 0 | 0 | 11 | 48 | 4 | 93 | 9 | | 30 |
| 165. | Orange juice (Citrus aurantiuni) | — | 98 | 0 | 0 | — | 2 | 9 | 2 | 180 | 12 | | 64 |
| 166. | Papaya, ripe (Carica papaya) | 75 | 91 | 1 | 0 | 1 | 7 | 32 | 6 | 69 | 11 | | 57 |
| 167. | Peaches (Amygdalus persica) | 88 | 86 | 1 | 0 | 1 | 10 | 50 | 2 | 453 | 21 | | 6 |
| 168. | Pears (Prunus persica) | 85 | 86 | 1 | 0 | 1 | 12 | 52 | 6 | 96 | 7 | | 0 |
| 169. | Pine apple (Ananas comosus) | 60 | 88 | 0 | 0 | 0 | 11 | 46 | 35 | 37 | 20 | | 39 |
| 170. | Plum (Prunus domestica) | 90 | 87 | 1 | 0 | 0 | 11 | 52 | 1 | 247 | 147 | | 5 |
| 171. | Pomegranate (Punica granatum) | 68 | 78 | 2 | 0 | 5 | 14 | 65 | 1 | 133 | 12 | | 16 |
| 172. | Pummelo (Citrus maxima) | — | 88 | 1 | 0 | 1 | 10 | 44 | | | | | 20 |
| 173. | Raisins (Vitis vinifera) | 100 | 20 | 2 | 0 | 1 | 75 | 308 | 52 | 860 | 42 | | 1 |

## TABLE H

### PROXIMATE PRINCIPLES, MINERALS AND VITAMINS
### VALUES PER 100 GMS OF EDIBLE PORTION

Na = Sodium
K = Pouassium
Mg = Magnesium

| S. No. | Name of foodstuff | Edible portion % | Moisture gm. | Protein gm. | Fat gm. | Fibre gm. | Carbo-hydrates gm. | Energy Kcal | Na mg | K mg | Mg mg | Cholesterol mg | Vitamin C mg |
|--------|-------------------|------------------|--------------|-------------|---------|-----------|--------------------|-------------|-------|------|-------|----------------|--------------|
| | | 1 | 2 | 3 | 4 | 5 | 6 | 7 | 8 | 9 | 10 | 11 | 12 |
| 174. | Sapota (Achras sapota) | 83 | 74 | 1 | 1 | 3 | 21 | 98 | 6 | 269 | 26 | | 6 |
| 175. | Seethaphal (Annona squamosa) | 45 | 70 | 2 | 0 | 3 | 23 | 104 | | 340 | 48 | | 37 |
| 176. | Strawberry (Fragaria vesca) | 96 | 88 | 1 | 0 | 1 | 10 | 44 | 2 | 160 | 12 | | 52 |
| 177. | Tomato, ripe (Lycopersicon esculentum) | 100 | 94 | 1 | 0 | 1 | 4 | 20 | 13 | 146 | 12 | | 27 |

## TABLE I
### PROXIMATE PRINCIPLES, MINERALS AND VITAMINS
### VALUES PER 100 GMS OF EDIBLE PORTION

Na = Sodium
K = Potassium
Mg = Magnesium

| S. No. | Name of foodstuff | Edible portion % | Moisture gm. | Protein gm. | Fat gm. | Fibre gm. | Carbo-hydrates gm. | Energy Kcal | Na mg | K mg | Mg mg | Cholesterol mg | Vitamin C mg |
|---|---|---|---|---|---|---|---|---|---|---|---|---|---|
| | | 1 | 2 | 3 | 4 | 5 | 6 | 7 | 8 | 9 | 10 | 11 | 12 |
| **FISHES AND OTHER SEA FOODS** | | | | | | | | | | | | | |
| 178. | Anchovy (Engraulis mystax) | 66 | 69 | 19 | 10 | — | 0 | 164 | | | | | |
| 179. | Bali kanakda, dried | — | 17 | 44 | 9 | — | 5 | 277 | | | | | — |
| 180. | Bele (Glassogobius giuris) | — | 80 | 14 | 1 | — | 3 | 75 | | | | | 3 |
| 181. | Bhetki, fresh (Lates calcarifer) | 50 | 80 | 15 | 1 | — | 3 | 79 | 66 | 173 | — | 40 | 10 |
| 182. | Bhetki, dried (Lates calcarifer) | — | 20 | 60 | 2 | — | 2 | 266 | | | | | |
| 183. | Blue mussel (Mytilus viridis) | 43 | 81 | 10 | 2 | — | 4 | 72 | | | | | |
| 184. | Bombay duck, dried (Harpodon neherens) | 75 | 17 | 62 | 4 | — | 2 | 293 | | | | | |
| 185. | Crab (muscle) (Paratelphusa spinigera) | — | 83 | 9 | 1 | — | 3 | 59 | 370 | 270 | 48 | | |
| 186. | Crab (small) | — | 65 | 11 | 10 | — | 9 | 169 | | | | 145 | — |
| 187. | Herring, Indian (Pellona brachysoma) | 50 | 73 | 20 | 3 | — | 2 | 119 | 67 | 340 | 29 | 75 | — |

TABLE I

PROXIMATE PRINCIPLES, MINERALS AND VITAMINS
VALUES PER 100 GMS OF EDIBLE PORTION

| S. No. | Name of foodstuff | Edible portion % | Moisture gm. | Protein gm. | Fat gm. | Fibre gm. | Carbo-hydrates gm. | Energy Kcal | Na mg | K mg | Mg mg | Cholesterol mg | Vitamin C mg |
|---|---|---|---|---|---|---|---|---|---|---|---|---|---|
| | | 1 | 2 | 3 | 4 | 5 | 6 | 7 | 8 | 9 | 10 | 11 | 12 |
| 188. | Hilsa (Clupea ilisha) | — | 54 | 22 | 19 | — | 3 | 273 | 52 | 183 | — | | 24 |
| 189. | Indian whiting (Sillago sihama) | 61 | 77 | 19 | 1 | — | 2 | 89 | 200 | 320 | 33 | | — |
| 190. | Katla (Catla catla) | — | 74 | 19 | 2 | — | 3 | 111 | 50 | 151 | — | | — |
| 191. | Lobster (Palaemon sp.) | — | 77 | 20 | 1 | — | 0 | 90 | 330 | 260 | 34 | 200 | — |
| 192. | Mackerel (Rastrelliger kanaguria) | 61 | 77 | 19 | 2 | — | 0 | 93 | 130 | 360 | 30 | 80 | — |
| 193. | Oil sardine (Sardinella longiceps) | 70 | 76 | 20 | 2 | — | 0 | 97 | | | | | — |
| 194. | Pomfrets, black (Formio niger) | 70 | 74 | 20 | 3 | — | 1 | 111 | | | | | — |
| 195. | Pomfrets, white (Stromateus sinensis) | 68 | 78 | 17 | 1 | — | 2 | 87 | | | | | 3 |
| 196. | Prawn (Penaeus sp.) | 45 | 77 | 19 | 1 | — | 1 | 89 | 66 | 262 | 42 | | — |
| 197. | Ravas (Polynemus tetradactylus) | 77 | 71 | 22 | 1 | — | 3 | 112 | | | | | — |

TABLE I

PROXIMATE PRINCIPLES, MINERALS AND VITAMINS
VALUES PER 100 GMS OF EDIBLE PORTION

Na = Sodium
K = Potassium
Mg = Magnesium

| S. No. | Name of foodstuff | Edible portion % | Moisture gm. | Protein gm. | Fat gm. | Fibre gm. | Carbo-hydrates gm. | Energy Kcal | Na mg | K mg | Mg mg | Cholesterol mg | Vitamin C mg |
|---|---|---|---|---|---|---|---|---|---|---|---|---|---|
| | | 1 | 2 | 3 | 4 | 5 | 6 | 7 | 8 | 9 | 10 | 11 | 12 |
| 198. | Rohu (Labeo rohita) | 78 | 77 | 17 | 1 | — | 4 | 97 | 101 | 288 | 13 | 11 | 12 |
| 199. | Sardine (Sardinella Filmbriata) | 60 | 78 | 21 | 2 | — | — | 101 | | | | | 22 |
| 200. | Shark (Carcharias sp.) | 67 | 76 | 22 | 0 | — | 1 | 93 | | | | 70 | — |
| | Oysters | | | | | | | | | | | | |
| | Tuna | | | | | | | | | | | | |
| 201. | Shrimp (small, dried) | — | 6 | 68 | 8 | — | — | 349 | 1260 | 130 | 35 | 200/161 | 65/51 |
| 202. | Sole (Ophiocephalus striatus) | — | 78 | 16 | 2 | — | 2 | 94 | — | — | — | 150 | 9 |

TABLE J

PROXIMATE PRINCIPLES, MINERALS AND VITAMINS
VALUES PER 100 GMS OF EDIBLE PORTION

K = Potassium
Mg = Magnesium

| S. No. | Name of foodstuff | Edible portion % | Moisture gm. | Protein gm. | Fat gm. | Fibre gm. | Carbo-hydrates gm. | Energy Kcal | Na mg | K mg | Mg mg | Cholesterol mg | Vitamin C mg |
|---|---|---|---|---|---|---|---|---|---|---|---|---|---|
| | | 1 | 2 | 3 | 4 | 5 | 6 | 7 | 8 | 9 | 10 | 11 | 12 |
| | OTHER FLESH FOODS | | | | | | | | | | | | |
| 203. | Beef muscle (Bos taurus) | — | 74 | 23 | 3 | — | — | 114 | 52 | 214 | 17 | 100 | 2 |
| 204. | Buffalo meat (Balbus bubalis) | — | 79 | 19 | 1 | — | — | 86 | | | | | — |
| 205. | Duck (Anas platyrayncha) | — | 72 | 22 | 5 | — | 0 | 130 | 110 | 290 | 19 | 70 | — |
| 206. | Egg, hen | — | 74 | 13 | 13 | — | — | 173 | 140 | 140 | 12 | 498 | 0 |
| 207. | Egg, turtle | — | 76 | 12 | 7 | — | 4 | 124 | | | | 70 | — |
| 208. | Goat meat | — | 74 | 21 | 4 | — | 1 | 118 | | | | 610 | 20 |
| 209. | Liver, sheep | — | 70 | 19 | 7 | — | — | 150 | 73 | 166 | — | 77 | |
| 210. | Mutton, muscle | — | 71 | 18 | 13 | — | — | 194 | 33 | 270 | — | 50 | |
| | Rabbit | | | | | | | | | | | 2000/ | |
| | Brain | | | | | | | | | | | 150 | |
| | Heart | | | | | | | | | | | 375 | |
| | Kidney | | | | | | | | | | | 250 | |
| | Pancreas | | | | | | | | | | | 110 | |
| 211. | Pigeon (Columbalivia intermedia) | — | 70 | 23 | 5 | — | — | 137 | | | | — | |
| 212. | Pork, muscle (Sus cristatus wagner) | — | 77 | 19 | 4 | — | — | 114 | 76 | 370 | 22 | 60 | 2 |

## TABLE K
### PROXIMATE PRINCIPLES, MINERALS AND VITAMINS
### VALUES PER 100 GMS OF EDIBLE PORTION

Na = Sodium
K = Potassium
Mg = Magnesium

| S. No. | Name of foodstuff | Edible portion % | Moisture gm. | Protein gm. | Fat gm. | Fibre gm. | Carbo-hydrates gm. | Energy Kcal | Na mg | K mg | Mg mg | Cholesterol mg | Vitamin C mg |
|---|---|---|---|---|---|---|---|---|---|---|---|---|---|
| | | 1 | 2 | 3 | 4 | 5 | 6 | 7 | 8 | 9 | 10 | 11 | 12 |
| **MILK AND DAIRY PRODUCTS** | | | | | | | | | | | | | |
| 213. | Milk, buffalo's | 100 | 81 | 4 | 9 | — | 5 | 117 | 19 | 90 | — | 11 | 1 |
| 214. | Milk, cow's | 100 | 87 | 3 | 4 | — | 4 | 67 | 16 | 140 | 12 | 14 | 2 |
| 215. | Milk, goat's | 100 | 87 | 3 | 4 | — | 5 | 72 | 11 | 110 | 20 | | 1 |
| 216. | Milk, human | 100 | 88 | 1 | 3 | — | 7 | 65 | | | | | 3 |
| 217. | Milk, ass's | 100 | 90 | 2 | 1 | — | 6 | 48 | 14 | 58 | 3 | 16 | 10 |
| 218. | Curds | 100 | 89 | 3 | 4 | — | 3 | 60 | 32 | 130 | — | | 1 |
| 219. | Butter milk | 100 | 97 | 1 | 1 | — | 0 | 15 | | | | | |
| 220. | Skimmed milk, liquid | 100 | 92 | 2 | 0. | — | 5 | 29 | | | | | 1 |
| 221. | Channa, cow's milk | 100 | 57 | 18 | 21 | — | 1 | 265 | | | | | 3 |
| 222. | Channa, buffalo milk | 100 | 54 | 13 | 23 | — | 8 | 292 | | | | | |
| 223. | Cheese | 100 | 40 | 24 | 25 | — | 6 | 348 | | | | 145 | |
| 224. | Kheer | 100 | 69 | 7 | 12 | — | 10 | 176 | | | | | 3 |
| 225. | Khoa (whole buffalo milk) | 100 | 31 | 15 | 31 | — | 20 | 421 | | | | | |
| 226. | Khoa (skimmed buffalo milk) | 100 | 46 | 22 | 2 | — | 26 | 206 | | | | | 1 |
| 227. | Khoa (whole cow milk) | 100 | 25 | 20 | 26 | — | 25 | 413 | | | | | 6 |
| 228. | Skimmed milk powder (cow's milk) | 100 | 4 | 38 | 0 | — | 51 | 357 | 532 | 1750 | | 1 | 5 |
| 229. | Whole milk powder (cow's milk) | 100 | 3 | 26 | 27 | — | 38 | 496 | | | | 88 | 4 |

## TABLE L

### PROXIMATE PRINCIPLES, MINERALS AND VITAMINS
### VALUES PER 100 GMS OF EDIBLE PORTION

Na = Sodium
K = Potassium
Mg = Magnesium

| S. No. | Name of foodstuff | Edible portion % | Moisture gm. | Protein gm. | Fat gm. | Fibre gm. | Carbo-hydrates gm. | Energy Kcal | Na mg | K mg | Mg mg | Cholesterol mg | Vitamin C mg |
|---|---|---|---|---|---|---|---|---|---|---|---|---|---|
| | | 1 | 2 | 3 | 4 | 5 | 6 | 7 | 8 | 9 | 10 | 11 | 12 |
| FATS AND EDIBLE OILS | | | | | | | | | | | | | |
| 230. | Butter | 100 | 19 | — | 81 | — | — | 729 | | | | 280 | — |
| 231. | Ghee (cow) | 100 | — | — | 100 | — | — | 900 | | | | 310 | — |
| 232. | Ghee (buffalo) | 100 | — | — | 100 | — | — | 900 | | | | | — |
| 233. | Hydrogenated oil (fortified) | 100 | — | — | 100 | — | — | 900 | | | | | |
| 234. | Cooking oil (Groundnut, Gingelly, Mustard, Coconut, etc.) | 100 | — | — | 100 | — | — | 900 | | | | | — |

Na = Sodium
K = Potassium
Mg = Magnesium

## TABLE M

### PROXIMATE PRINCIPLES, MINERALS AND VITAMINS
### VALUES PER 100 GMS OF EDIBLE PORTION

| S. No. | Name of foodstuff | Edible portion % | Moisture gm. | Protein gm. | Fat gm. | Fibre gm. | Carbo-hydrates gm. | Energy Kcal | Na mg | K mg | Mg mg | Cholesterol mg | Vitamin C mg |
|---|---|---|---|---|---|---|---|---|---|---|---|---|---|
| | | 1 | 2 | 3 | 4 | 5 | 6 | 7 | 8 | 9 | 10 | 11 | 12 |
| | **MISCELLANEOUS FOODSTUFFS** | | | | | | | | | | | | |
| 235. | Arrow root flour (Maranta arundinacea) | — | 16 | 0 | 0 | — | 83 | 334 | 3 | 20 | — | | 12 |
| 236. | Bajjar bhang (Piper betle) | — | 7 | 17 | 8 | 2 | 62 | 392 | — | — | 405 | | 0 |
| 237. | Betel leaves (Piper betle) | — | 85 | 3 | 1 | 2 | 6 | 44 | | | | | 5 |
| 238. | Biscuits, salt | 100 | 4 | 7 | 32 | — | 55 | 534 | | | | | |
| 239. | Biscuits, sweet | 100 | 5 | 6 | 15 | — | 72 | 450 | | | | — | |
| 240. | Bread, brown | 100 | 39 | 9 | 1 | 1 | 49 | 244 | | | | — | |
| 241. | Bread, white | 100 | 39 | 8 | 1 | 0 | 52 | 245 | | | | — | |
| 242. | Cane sugar (Saccharum officinarum) | 100 | 0 | 0 | 0 | 0 | 99 | 398 | | | | | |
| 243. | Coconut, tender (Cocos nucifera) | — | 91 | 1 | 1 | — | 6 | 41 | | | | | — |
| 244. | Coconut milk (Cocos nucifera) | 100 | 43 | 3 | 41 | 0 | 12 | 430 | | | | | — |
| 245. | Coconut water | 100 | 94 | 1 | 0 | 0 | 4 | 24 | 10 | 295 | 50 | | 2 |
| 246. | Fish liver oil | 100 | — | — | 100 | — | — | 900 | | | | — | 3 |
| 247. | Honey | — | 21 | 0 | 0 | — | 79 | 319 | | | | — | 2 |
| 248. | Jaggery (cane) | — | 4 | 0 | 0 | — | 95 | 383 | | | | | 4 |
| 249. | Makhana (Euryale ferox) | — | 13 | 10 | 0 | — | 77 | 347 | | | | | 0 |

Na = Sodium
K = Potassium
Mg = Magnesium

## TABLE M
### PROXIMATE PRINCIPLES, MINERALS AND VITAMINS
#### VALUES PER 100 GMS OF EDIBLE PORTION

| S. No. | Name of foodstuff | Edible portion % | Moisture gm. | Protein gm. | Fat gm. | Fibre gm. | Carbo hydrates gm. | Energy Kcal | Na mg | K mg | Mg mg | Cholesterol mg | Vitamin C mg |
|---|---|---|---|---|---|---|---|---|---|---|---|---|---|
| | | 1 | 2 | 3 | 4 | 5 | 6 | 7 | 8 | 9 | 10 | 11 | 12 |
| 251. | Pappad | 100 | 20 | 19 | 0 | — | 52 | 288 | | | | | 0 |
| 252. | Sago | — | 12 | 0 | 0 | — | 87 | 351 | | | | | — |
| 253. | Sugar cane juice . | — | 90 | 0 | 0 | — | 9 | 39 | | | | | — |
| 254. | Toddy, fermented | — | 98 | 0 | 0 | — | 2 | 8 | | | | | — |
| 255. | Toddy, sweet | — | 85 | 0 | 0 | — | 14 | 59 | | | | | — |
| 256. | Yeast, dried (Brewer's) | — | 14 | 39 | 1 | 0 | 39 | 320 | | | | | 0 |

## DISTILLED ALCOHOLIC BEVERAGES

| 1) Distilled spirits, liquors or spirits | | Usual portion in ml. | Approximate alcohol by volume | Approximate calorie value of usual portion | Approximate calorie value of 100 ml. |
|---|---|---|---|---|---|
| | | | 1 G. of Alcohol (about 1.16 ml.) = 7.1 cal | | |
| Brandy | Indian | 20 | 43 | 61 | 306 |
| | Foreign | 20 | 52 | 73 | 365 |
| Gin | Indian | 50 | 43 | 164 | 327 |
| | | 43 | 43 | 141 | 327 |
| | Foreign | 50 | 80 | 295 | 590 |
| | | 43 | 80 | 254 | 590 |
| Rum | Indian | 50 | 43 | 154 | 307 |
| | | 43 | 43 | 132 | 307 |
| | Foreign | 50 | Varies | | |
| Vodka | Indian | 30 | 40 | 85 | 284 |
| | Foreign | 30 | 48 | 102 | 341 |
| Whisky | Indian | 50 | 43 | 153 | 305 |
| | Foreign | 50 | 50 | 178 | 355 |

| Liqueurs, or Cordials, coloured, flavoured and sugared (not less than 2.5% sugar) | Usual portion in ml. | Approximate alcohol by volume | Approximate calorie value of usual portion | Approximate calorie value of 100 ml. |
|---|---|---|---|---|
| Anisette | 20 | 27 | 42 | 208 |
| Apricot | 20 | 30 | 67 | 333 |
| Blackberry | 20 | 30 | 67 | 335 |
| Cherry | 20 | 31 | 68 | 342 |
| Creme de Cacao | 20 | 26 | 61 | 307 |
| Curacao | 20 | 36 | 76 | 378 |
| Kummel | 20 | 43 | 85 | 425 |
| Maraschino | 20 | 31 | 68 | 342 |
| Peach | 20 | 38 | 78 | 392 |
| Prunelle | 20 | 40 | 81 | 406 |
| Sloe gin | 20 | 30 | 67 | 335 |
| Triple sce | 20 | 39 | 80 | 399 |
| The proprietary brands | | | | |
| are Benedictine | 20 | '43 | 89 | 445 |
| Chartreuse, green | ·20 | 55 | 106 | 531 |
| yellow | 20 | 43 | 89 | 445 |

Liqueurs or Cordials, contd.

| | Usual portion in ml. | Approximate alcohol by volume | Approximate calorie value of usual portion | Approximate calorie value of 100 ml. |
|---|---|---|---|---|
| Cherry Heering | 20 | 25 | 58 | 290 |
| Cointreau | 20 | 40 | 81 | 406 |
| Drambuie | 20 | 40 | 81 | 406 |
| Grand Marnier | 20 | 40 | 81 | 406 |
| Irish Mist | 20 | 40 | 81 | 406 |
| Tia Maria (coffee) | 20 | 32 | 70 | 349 |

## TABLE O

### WINES

| 1) Still or natural wines | Usual portion in ml. | Approximate alcohol by volume | Approximate calorie value of usual portion | Approximate calorie value of 100 ml. |
|---|---|---|---|---|
| Red | 120 | 11 | 108 | 90 |
| Rose | 120 | 11 | 108 | 90 |
| White | 120 | 10 | 100 | 83 |
| **2) Fortified and Aromatic Wines** | | | | |
| Port | 30 | 19 | 55 | 183 |
| Sherry, dry | 30 | 18 | 43 | 144 |
| Sherry, sweet | 30 | 18 | 45 | 150 |
| Vermouth | 105 | 19 | 169 | 161 |
| **3) Sparkling Wines** | | | | |
| Champagne | 135 | 12 | 124 | 92 |

TABLE P

**FERMENTED MALT BEVERAGES**

| eer or ale, lager | | | | |
|---|---|---|---|---|
| eer, brown | 250 | 3 | 100 | 40 |
| eer, strong | 250 | 7 | 195 | 78 |
| oddy | 250 | 4 (1 to 7) | 143 | 67 |

(Calories vary, depending on alcohol content and natural sugars. Vitamins $B_1$, $B_7$ and C are also present in toddy)

weet bottled drinks, e.g. Cola (various types). Orange, Pineapple, etc. contain 5-80 calories/bottle (200-250 ml.). Mangola contains 140 calories/bottle.

# OXALIC ACID CONTENT

### Food stuffs with Oxalic Acid content more than 100 mg per 100 gm

This may be of importance to patients with tendency for Renal Stones.

| Name of the food-stuff | Oxalic Ac mg per 100 gr |
| --- | --- |
| 1. Almond (Badam) | |
| 2. Amaranth tender (Math) | 4 |
| 3. Amla (Awla) | 7 |
| 4. Bhangari | 2 |
| 5. Cashew nuts (Kaju) | 12 |
| 6. Chookri Ka atta | 31 |
| 7. Chookri Ka Patta | 14 |
| 8. Cucumber (Kakadi) | 622 |
| 9. Curry leaves (Kandhi Limb Patta) | 10 |
| 10. Drum stick leaves (Shevgyachi Pane) | 13 |
| 11. Garden Cress Seeds (Methi) | 10 |
| 12. Gingelly seeds (Til) | 14 |
| 13. Gogu (Ambadi) | 170 |
| 14. Horse gram dal (Kuleeth) | 14 |
| 15. Khesari dal (Lakhdal) | 41 |
| 16. Lotus stem (Kamal Ka Danda) | 12 |
| 17. Neem Leaves (Tender) (Mitha Limbda) | 42 |
| 18. Paruppu Keerai (Padwal leaves) | 15 |
| 19. Phalsa | 167 |
| 20. Plantain flower (Kelphool) | 20 |
| 21. Plantain Green (Kacha Kela) | 42 |
| 22. Spinach (Palak) | 48 |
| 23. Tamarind leaves (Tender) (Imli Ke Patte) | 658 |
| 24. Wood apple (Kawath) | 196 |
| | 272 |

## TABLE R

## PURINE CONTENT OF FOOD

When you have Gout or high uric acid, watch for purine content of your diet.

| Not allowed—High 150-800 mg./100 gm. | Medium. One serving/day 50-150 mg./100 gm. | Unlimited—low 0-15 mg./100 gm. |
|---|---|---|
| Sweet breads | Meat | Vegetables |
| Sardines | Fish | Fruit |
| Liver | Seafoods | Milk |
| Kidneys | Peas | Cheese |
| Meat extract | Beans | Eggs |
| | Lentils | Cereals |
| | Asparagus | |
| | Cauliflower | |
| | Spinach | |
| | Mushroom | |

# DESIRABLE WEIGHTS FOR MEN
## (Aged 40 And Over)

| HEIGHT | | WEIGHT* Medium Frame | |
| Centimeters | Inches | Kilos | Pounds |
|---|---|---|---|
| 150 | 59.1 | 51 | 112.4 |
| 152 | 59.8 | 52 | 114.0 |
| 154 | 60.6 | 54 | 119.0 |
| 156 | 61.4 | 55 | 121.3 |
| 158 | 62.2 | 56 | 123.5 |
| 160 | 63.0 | 57 | 125.7 |
| 162 | 63.8 | 59 | 130.1 |
| 164 | 64.6 | 60 | 132.3 |
| 166 | 65.4 | 62 | 136.7 |
| 168 | 66.1 | 63 | 138.9 |
| 170 | 66.9 | 65 | 143.3 |
| 172 | 67.7 | 67 | 147.7 |
| 174 | 68.5 | 68 | 149.9 |
| 176 | 69.3 | 70 | 154.3 |
| 178 | 70.1 | 72 | 158.7 |
| 180 | 70.9 | 74 | 163.1 |
| 182 | 71.7 | 76 | 167.6 |
| 184 | 72.4 | 77 | 169.8 |
| 186 | 73.2 | 78 | 172.0 |
| 188 | 74.0 | 80 | 176.4 |
| 190 | 74.8 | 81 | 178.6 |

* Weight as ordinarily dressed. For small frame deduct 10% and large frame add 10%.

For women deduct 2 cm from the actual height and then read off the weight from the above chart.

Under the age of 40, deduct approximately 3% for every 5 years.

# INDEX